miserably happy

miserably happy

Infuse Your Life with Genuine Meaning, Purpose, Health, and Happiness

Dr. Kevin Brannick
PsyD, MA

—and—

Dr. Michelle A. Brannick
ND, DC

New York

miserably happy
Infuse Your Life with Genuine Meaning, Purpose, Health, and Happiness

Published in New York, New York, by Morgan James Publishing. Morgan James and The Entrepreneurial Publisher are trademarks of Morgan James, LLC.
www.MorganJamesPublishing.com

The Morgan James Speakers Group can bring authors to your live event. For more information or to book an event visit The Morgan James Speakers Group at
www.TheMorganJamesSpeakersGroup.com.

bitlit

A **free** eBook edition is available
with the purchase of this print book.

CLEARLY PRINT YOUR NAME ABOVE IN UPPER CASE

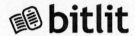

Instructions to claim your free eBook edition:
1. Download the BitLit app for Android or iOS
2. Write your name in **UPPER CASE** on the line
3. Use the BitLit app to submit a photo
4. Download your eBook to any device

ISBN 978-1-63047-645-8 paperback
ISBN 978-1-63047-645-8 eBook
Library of Congress Control Number:
2015939861

Cover Design by:
Rachel Lopez
www.r2cdesign.com

Interior Design by:
Bonnie Bushman
The Whole Caboodle Graphic Design

In an effort to support local communities and raise awareness and funds, Morgan James Publishing donates a percentage of all book sales for the life of each book to Habitat for Humanity Peninsula and Greater Williamsburg.

Get involved today, visit
www.MorganJamesBuilds.com

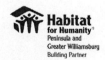

Habitat
for Humanity
Peninsula and
Greater Williamsburg
Building Partner

To:
Yeats and Brendan

Table of Contents

acknowledgements

We could not and would not have written this book without the support, love, and presence of our two sons, Yeats and Brendan. Human beings cannot thrive or even survive without being connected to other human beings. Clearly, the most profound connection we human beings have is our connection to our children.

This book also drew inspiration and wisdom from our patients. Working hand-in-hand with our patients provides us with a bottomless well of energy and an ever-deepening experience of the meaning and purpose of life.

Through our family, friends, patients, and community we have discovered that the meaning and purpose of life is ultimately determined by the quality and sustainability of our relationships. The quality and sustainability of our relationships to ourselves, others, our communities and our planet, is the exclusive currency of genuine happiness.

This book was written with the hope that it will, in some small way, leave behind a more humanized world for our world community and future generations to come.

miserable-happy
symptoms and underlying cause

Indeed, man wishes to be happy even when he so lives as to make happiness impossible.

—St. Augustine

Our nation is in the grip of a severe health care crisis which fuels and sustains our seemingly endless financial crisis. Both crises are complicated by our politicians. Our political leaders, who are elected to serve all of us "we the people" instead pander to the extreme elements of their parties fearing that special interest groups will run them out of office if they act reasonably and responsibly. All three crises are symptoms of a much deeper and more pervasive problem. The underlying cause of our troubles is our indiscriminate pursuit of happiness. Our indiscriminate pursuit of happiness obscures our sense of what is reasonable and responsible. Our desire to be happy, happy, happy is leading us down a path that can only end in our becoming more miserable than Pinocchio became as he was morphing into a happy, happy, happy Jackass on Pleasure Island.

Our obsession with happiness has an addictive quality. Our relentless search for our next happiness fix fuels Madison Avenue, which sells all its wares based on the promise of delivering the happiness we so desperately seek and believe we are entitled to. Our addiction to pursuing happiness is apparent by the fact that, as of this writing, there were 42 titles on Amazon that claim to hold the secret to happiness. Moreover, happiness road map books are usually at the top of the New York Times Best Seller list. There are also thousands of Internet sites and articles that claim to have a pill or a process that is certain to make us happy 24/7. Lastly, the pharmaceutical industry markets and sells over 279 billion dollars' worth of drugs all based on explicit and implicit claims that the drugs will not only protect us from the unhappiness of illness and death, they will turn our lives into happy walks on the beach. Most of these drugs and virtually every other legally addictive "happy" product sold on the corner of "happy and healthy" will lead us to the misery and despair of skid row if they don't kill us first. In reality the happy market has a lot more in common with Pinocchio's journey to Pleasure Island than with health and genuine happiness.

Our book takes a different approach. Our book will confirm that we humans have the capacity to live deeply meaningful and genuinely happy lives without the happy pills, happy sugar drenched, happy additive filled, and happy GMO'd products, happy "secrets," and happy egocentric me, me, me guidelines that are in reality discussing excuses for healthcare treatments, food, and Pleasure Island utopías. Our book will also offer an invaluable, yet non-prescriptive, path to health and genuine happiness. Our book will argue that the counterweight to Pinocchio's Pleasure Island happiness is reasonable and responsible action. Reasonable and responsible action, while often accompanied by discomfort and the sacrifice of the immediate experience of pleasure, is our exclusive path to health and genuine happiness. Moreover, as will be shown, reasonable and responsible action is the essence of both our DNA and spirituality.

Our book will not anchor its argument on concepts or guidelines that might define reasonable and responsible behavior. Instead, this book will identify the fixed laws and patterns of biology which, moment to moment, seek optimal health by pursuing, grasping, and sustaining healthy connections which are nature's inbuilt demands for reasonable and responsible action. Optimal connectedness to ourselves, others, and our environment, irrespective of our emotional experience—pleasant or painful—defines genuine happiness. Thus, if we shift our focus from Pleasure Island happiness to achieving optimal connectedness through reasonable and responsible action we can eliminate our political gridlock, solve both our healthcare and financial crises, clean up our life-sustaining planet, and create a culture of genuine happiness.

The path to genuine happiness has little to do with our common beliefs about happiness. In fact, as will be shown, our common beliefs and experiences of happiness are the primary cause of our fall from the mountaintop of genuine meaning and purpose into the dark and lonely canyon of misery and despair.

As indicated above, in presenting an invulnerable path to genuine happiness we will not offer a series of exercises or prescribed daily activities or "to do lists" as a path to happiness. Such formulas for happiness are counter-productive and are doomed to fail because they do not, and cannot, consider the unique make-up of our individual life and the circumstances of our moment-to-moment situations. Moreover, the bulk of such formulaic approaches to happiness base their claims on sentimental and ill-defined or undefined concepts of what it means to be human. For example, authors often claim that human happiness is based on some unexplained spiritual entity that exists outside of us. They often suggest our spirit is not human. They claim that while our "mystery" spirit is within us, it is not part of us. Thus, we are told to ultimately base our lives on an undefined and unknowable "spirit" that plays a critical role in our experience of happiness. We are led to believe we can plug into this unknown "spirit" or energy, which will provide us with a happiness utopia for no discernible reason. However, the great spiritual leader Thomas Merton cautioned us about such assumptions of happiness fearing that what we perceive as good might indeed be evil. In other words, relying on an unknown spirit or energy as the source of happiness often becomes a quicksand pit of misery and despair. Others offer "magic" pills, herbs, or prescriptive lifestyles. Rarely is there any attempt to ground these claims and any foundational understanding of what it is to be human or the basic demands of the biology from which we humans have emerged.

Currently, religion, self-proclaimed happiness gurus, and evidence-based "scientists" ground human happiness on their dogmatic beliefs rather than comprehensive and systematic research data. Science demands comprehensive data and a systematic understanding of data to achieve a close approximation of the phenomenon being studied. Religions rely on dogmatic beliefs about God, prophets, scripture, or tradition rather than science in determining the reality of human happiness. Happiness gurus typically rely on some unexplained claim of a "vital force," "universe energy," "secret," or hide behind some other bait that can't be proved or disproved rather than science to sell their claims of human happiness. Evidence-based "scientists" rely on the completely and utterly discredited notion that human science must be restricted to observable data to sells their claims of happiness pills, procedures, and products. Evidence-based human "science" is dogma not science. Evidence-based research, by deliberately excluding that data of our non-observable mental properties is not comprehensive.

Evidence-based human research is simply the statistical manipulation of material-only data masquerading as science. Evidence-based research, while producing trillions of dollars for its profiteers, is an emperor with no clothes that now kills close to a million people a year, eats up 20% of our GDP, causes 62-70% of personal bankruptcies, creates superbugs, and inflicts massive environmental pollution on our planet.

Herein loom some critical questions, such as "what is this spiritual force, energy, or agent?" "What if there is no spiritual force, energy, or agent?" "If such a force, energy, or agent does exist, what if it is an anti-happiness force, energy, or agent?" These elephants in the room issues are denied, masked, or suppressed for no apparent reason other than they upset the happiness profit machine applecart. However, if such a spiritual source does exist, it is possible that it has absolutely no interest in our happiness whatsoever and, in fact, may punish our pursuit of pleasure-based happiness. Thus, the reasonable and responsible course of action would be to identify whether or not such a happiness source, energy, or agent actually exists. If it does exist we can then try to determine how it actually supports or diminishes our experience of happiness. In the meantime, it is unreasonable and irresponsible to make claims about something we can conceive of, but can't comprehend or validate. Such unverified claims are little more than magical thinking, and recommendations based on such claims run the risk of causing more misery and despair than the sought after happiness outcomes. From a professional standpoint and in virtually any regulated industry, making claims about the unknown is considered malpractice or illegal. However, in peddling spirit-based happiness snake oil and happiness in general, it is buyer beware.

This book will break with the vast majority of happiness manuals, prophets, and products by providing precise definitions of our human make-up: body-mind-spirit. These definitions are open to scientific verification and represent a quantum leap in our innate demand for a reasonable and responsible explanation of what it is to be human and how humans can come to experience genuine happiness.

To this end, Chapter 2 will provide a brief history of happiness and propose an understanding of happiness that recognizes both the positive and negative dimensions of happiness. We will discuss how the negative dimension of happiness results in the preponderance of human suffering. I will also discuss how positive happiness is at the core of human nature and determines the meaning and purpose of human life.

Chapter 3 will provide an overview of our evidence-based conventional medicine system. While necessarily technical, the presentation is essential in understanding how our culture is being evidence-based into mental, spiritual, economic, and environmental misery.

Chapter 4 will provide an overview of naturopathic medicine, a comprehensive primary care medical system that can overcome the challenges of the evidence-based conventional medicine system. It will be shown how naturopathic medicine works with our body-mind-spirit dramatically increasing the possibility of preventing illness, supporting body-mind-spirit health and wellness, and supporting genuine human happiness.

Chapter 5 will provide an overview of emergent property theory, which provides a scientific explanation of our body-mind-spirit. Again, while technical, the overview of emergent property theory will provide a solution to the core challenges we face in our personal lives, our communities, our nation, and the world, by giving both a scientific explanation and methodology for understanding the human body-mind-spirit. Thus, we will provide a definitive understanding of human meaning, purpose, and genuine happiness.

Chapter 6 will provide some concluding thoughts. It will be shown that the normal functioning of our body-mind-spirit determines what genuine happiness is and what role genuine happiness plays in the genuine meaning and purpose of human life. It will be shown that genuine happiness is often a humbling byproduct of selfless service to others. Moreover, it will be shown that genuine happiness often emerges when we embrace the discomfort of reasonable and responsible actions and patterns. It will also be shown that Pleasure Island happiness is not only destructive to our body-mind-spirit, it is destructive to our relationships, our communities, and our planet.

At our clinics we see firsthand how addictive and destructive the pursuit of Pleasure Island happiness can be. At the beginning of virtually every first office visit our patients, in a rather sobering manner, say in one way or another, that they have come to the clinic because they are "not happy." Our response is to tell them that their unhappiness is their best friend. It is telling them that something is out of balance. Moreover, by the fact that they know they are unhappy they have begun to mine their critical body-mind-spirit data to meet whatever challenges they may face. We often, based on the specific patient's situation, tell them that their unhappiness is a blunt message confirming that the meaning and purpose of life is not happiness or the pursuit of happiness. We tell them that every genuine impulse in our body-mind-spirit has two aspirations- neither of which are the attainment of pleasure-based happiness. The first is to seek the reasonable. The second is to act responsibly. By seeking the reasonable and choosing to act in accordance with what they determine to be reasonable or, in and other words, to act responsibly, they become deeply connected to themselves, others and, indeed, the universe. In other words, our body-mind-spirit is our source of wisdom or knowing the right path of action to take and our capacity for integrity, which is to act in accordance with what we know to be reasonable.

The reasonable and responsible governs nature's innate impulse to create healthy connections. Your body-mind-spirit is engaged in the process now. You are questioning whether or not what you are reading makes sense. Through your questioning, you will either reach a reasonable understanding of what you are reading or realize you need additional information. Unless you obstruct it, your body-mind-spirit relentlessly pursues the reasonable. Responsible action is simply to act in accordance with what you know to be reasonable. The objective of biology is to secure healthy connections and healthy connections are created and sustained by reasonable and responsible activities. Reasonable and responsible activities are activities that embrace biology's innate laws and patterns. Both concepts, reasonable and responsible, will be precisely defined and discussed in Chapter 6.

In short, we tell our patients that the meaning and purpose of life is to live within the nature of our body-mind-spirit which demands reasonable and responsible action, moment-to-moment, irrespective of emotional, physical, financial, or any other consequences. For example, most, if not all, genuine religious prophets and heroes are prophets and heroes because of the sacrifices they made and suffering they endured in pursuit of what they knew was a reasonable and responsible response to whatever challenge they faced. We all know the permanent satisfaction we experience as the result of any uncomfortable, or even painful, reasonable and responsible action we've taken. For example, as any parent, caregiver, or person who has ever been responsible for the welfare of others knows, reasonable and responsible care is not concerned with the caregiver's happiness. We don't give a child candy or let them engage in dangerous activities so they will be pacified and we will be happy. Caregiving is about creating reasonable and responsible relationship patterns in our children, which instills a deep sense of secure attachment. Such secure attachments deepen the experience of connectedness, which is the hallmark of meaningful, sustainable, and healthy relationships, that is, genuine happiness.

The reasonable and responsible is not interested in happiness, but instead is focused on operating within the reality of the biological laws that connect all aspects of the natural universe in a healthy and sustainable unity.

Happiness, genuine happiness, as it turns out, is realized through the ever-deepening sense of connectedness we realize through our body-mind-spirit properties. When we embrace the activity of being reasonable and responsible, moment-to-moment, we experience genuine happiness.

P is an example of a patient who realized the power and strength of her body-mind-spirit by following through on what she knew would be an uncomfortable but reasonable and responsible course of action to protect her children and herself from potential danger. P came to us just after leaving an abusive partner. She was emotionally and physically hurt by the relationship, but knew she had to get out of the relationship to protect her two children. P was unsure of herself, anxious, and in need of support. She was adjusting to her failed relationship and also needed help with nutrition, sleep, and emotional and physical exhaustion. While uncomfortable with engaging in the legal process, she sought and received legal protection. She also reached out to her family, friends, and community support systems. Additionally, based on blood work and lab tests she changed her diet. Together, her actions enabled her to tap into her vast inner reservoir of energy which allowed her to experience a deep sense of peace knowing that, while uncomfortable and painful, she was facing her challenges in a reasonable and responsible manner. She knew she would have no regrets about her course of action and that she was experiencing and developing an effective pattern of dealing with any future challenges she might face. She was deeply satisfied that she was successfully working through her adversity without having to take any "happy" pills that would mask her need to take the painful actions she needed to take, potentially harm her health, leave her with significant medical bills, and reduce her capacity to experience and learn effective problem-solving processes.

We provided her with a nutritional plan, supplements to replace nutritional deficiencies and counseling to gain insight into her anxiety.

Within two months she was eating a much healthier diet, taking care of herself, and her energy and mental clarity increased dramatically. Her sleep was improving, muscle cramps resolved, and her periods returned. Counseling gave her a sense of feeling understood and feeling connected to herself, her children, and her community.

P is a wonderful example of how treating the whole person, mind-body-spirit can change a life. She is now completing her master's degree and her family is adjusting well to a new, healthier life. The whole is always greater than, and qualitatively different than, the sum of its parts; as P became stronger mentally and spiritually she became stronger physically. Anxiety was not the enemy to be suppressed with a pill. Her anxiety made her aware that something was wrong and gave her the motivation, strength, and energy to make the changes she knew she had to make irrespective of how uncomfortable it was. As a result she gained self-confidence in both her personal and professional lives.

As in P's experience, the key to resolving the underlying issues that plague humanity is understanding the human body-mind-spirit and how our body-mind-spirit enables us, through our consciousness, to make sense of our world and determine what is a reasonable and responsible course of action, moment-to-moment. It is precisely the sum of our body-mind-spirit that enables us to experience and act in accordance with our capacity to understand the reasonable and subsequently act responsibly. Whether or not the reasonable and responsible makes us comfortable or uncomfortable is not the concern. Reasonable and responsible living, moment-to-moment, is the bedrock of health and the source of creating a meaningful and genuinely happy life.

Our health and wellness are based, not on our experience of happiness, but on our commitment to reasonable and responsible activity. The meaning and purpose of human life is the ever-deepening experience of connectedness realized through embracing our created capacity to act reasonably and responsibly moment-to-moment. To the extent we live our lives in such a manner we participate in and become ever more deeply connected to the source of all that is reasonable and responsible, genuine and authentic, true and good. Creating healthy connections is built into our DNA and is the core demand of our body-mind-spirit.

Given the centrality of our body-mind-spirit in creating and connecting us to genuine meaning and purpose, we ask our patients to think about where they believe they are on the wellness continuum which runs from opposing poles of alienation and connectedness. We next ask them why they think they are in that place. Their task, we suggest, is to make whatever changes are necessary to move toward the connectedness pole of the continuum. This involves each patient making changes in one or more areas of their life. We cannot, and do not, offer a cookie cutter approach. Each patient is unique and demands an approach that respects the totality of their life. Each patient has needs involving, but not limited to diet, exercise, sleep, relationships, habits, life history, and their decision-making processes. All such activities are paramount in creating and implementing a reasonable and responsible treatment plan.

In working with patients we affirm what they already know. They know they need to take a detailed look at their lifestyle and decision-making process. They know they need to make some changes. They know that they need to continue the work they've already begun in moving toward lifestyle patterns and decision-making processes, which will deepen their connectedness. We affirm that over the course of each day we all make hundreds of choices. We affirm that while we might like to imagine ourselves in any number of ways, we are simply the sum of the choices we make. There is no such thing as a higher-self waiting for actualization. We change for the better when we commit ourselves to a pattern of making reasonable and responsible choices. We are our choices. It is that simple, and while it might, at times, be uncomfortable or even painful, it is the exclusive path to genuine happiness.

Thus, we discuss how, over the course of a day, the demands of reasonable and responsible choices require us to sacrifice momentary experiences of pleasure or comfort and embrace the discomfort often associated with the genuine happiness that emerges from reasonable and responsible choices and activity. We refer to the contrast in these choices as, "The Twinkie Dilemma."

the twinkie dilemma

The Twinkie Dilemma captures the fact that every thought we have and act upon to satisfy an unreasonable and irresponsible desire or craving, such as the consumption of junk food, activates a number of physical and mental responses that produce the experience of "pleasure happiness." If we engage in such activity we harm our body-mind-spirit. Given that our choices define who we are, we ask our patients to recall a recent Twinkie Dilemma event they experienced.

We then ask them to report how they presently feel about the choice they made. Generally, they report being unhappy and self-alienated if they chose to "eat the Twinkie." Their experience of self-alienation generally has a negative effect on their relationships with others. They move towards the alienation pole of the wellness continuum. If they chose not to "eat the Twinkie" they feel empowered, they feel good about themselves, and their positive self-image has a beneficial effect on their relationships with others. They move toward the connected pole on the wellness continuum. Wellness, as it turns out, is not determined by an emotional state or physical condition, but instead is ultimately determined by where we are on the alienation-connectedness continuum based on the sum of our decisions.

"Symptoms" such as sadness, anger, anxiety, weight gain, back pain, headaches, and many other physical and mental complaints or conditions are, in most circumstances, simply biological messages that direct us to take responsible action based on our ability to come to a reasonable understanding of whatever we are attending to. If we seek the information we need to make reasonable decisions, and then implement what we know is reasonable, we deepen our experience of ourselves, we enhance our capacity to help others and nurture our planet. In sum, we participate more fully in the connectedness of the entire universe of being. We cannot change if we take a pill that masks, suppresses, or destroys our body-mind-spirit messaging. Masking or suppressing the symptoms is shooting the messenger.

E is an example of how we can win our daily Twinkie Dilemma battles.

E, a 55-year-old man, who was diagnosed with diabetes type 2 in 2002 and has been on medications since, is a great example of how to achieve a successful outcome of the Twinkie Dilemma. E did not like the side effects of his medications. He did not like how he felt and the medications were not doing much to help him, so he stopped his medications a week before coming to our clinic. He wanted a more natural approach to help him regulate his sugar. His sugar readings were between 100-200 and were unstable.

We worked to improve his diet and recommended some supplements and exercises to reduce and stabilize his sugar. Within three weeks his sugar was stabilizing with readings averaging 120 and he felt much better with increased energy. Additionally, his clothes felt looser and he felt decreased inflammation. The rash on his arms, which he had for years, started to resolve. His blood pressure also decreased from 144/80 to 130/80.

After nine weeks of adhering to his new reasonable and responsible lifestyle, his sugar levels continued to decrease along with additional weight loss. When I asked him about his ability to adhere to the treatment plan his answer was simply, "I wanted to get my health back and would do anything for it. If that means I can't eat something, so be it. It is not worth the damage that eating the wrong thing does. You only end up cheating yourself." It was E's attitude and dedication to lifestyle changes that helped him win his daily Twinkie Dilemma battles and achieve the genuine happiness of health and vitality.

pleasure island misery and despair

Often our movement toward the alienation pole of the wellness continuum results from our distorted idea of happiness. While happiness has always been a core human interest, it is quite possibly the most misunderstood of all human experiences. Our interest in happiness is due to the fact that happiness is a powerful emotion. In fact, happiness might well be our emotional baseline. Given the central role happiness plays in our daily lives, it is not surprising that happiness is one of the most researched and written about topics in both scientific and popular circles. However, while happiness, and the pursuit of happiness, is universally viewed as positive, our experience of happiness, as argued above, often leads to misery and despair.

The consequences of happiness are often lost in ideals and aspirations to be happy. In our often-blind desire to be happy we minimize or deny the known consequences of our attempts to attain happiness by misplacing the source of our unhappiness. We seek strategies to change family members, friends, co-workers, institutions, God, and just about anything we can think of to remove obstacles we believe are blocking our path to happiness. We reach for medications, abuse all kinds of substances, and engage in all kinds of activities that mask and suppress our discomfort. Once in a blue moon we attempt to gain insight into why we are placing obstacles in our path to genuine happiness. However, when we reflect on our choices we often come to realize that our unhappiness comes from our pursuit of Pleasure

Island happiness and we come to realize it is this pursuit that has left us feeling miserable.

On the positive side, our desire to experience happiness, often at any cost, can transcend our moment-to-moment challenges providing the fuel that drives us to overcome hardships and heartaches and can also sustain us as we strive to meet daily challenges or accomplish great things. Moreover, as we strive to realize our dreams, we can inspire others to pursue their dreams. The trick is to understand the difference between gratuitous pleasure-based happiness and reasonable- and responsible-based genuine happiness.

defining happiness

Given the central role happiness plays in our lives and in shaping human history, it would seem that happiness would be a relatively simple concept to grasp. You would think that defining and learning how to be happy would be as easy as walking and chewing gum at the same time. However, defining and attaining happiness seems to get more complicated as our experience and knowledge increases. Thus, while attempts to define happiness and create happiness paths are as old as human existence, our understanding of happiness remains an enigma wrapped in a riddle. For example, in a BBC news article from 2006, Dr. Morten L. Kringelbach states that, "for thousands of years people have pursued happiness, but the problem has been that it has always been seen as a kind of fuzzy concept."[1]

Happiness means different things to different people. One person's experience of happiness can be another person's experience of fear, anxiety, or sadness. For example, while rock climbing makes some happy, others can feel anxiety by simply looking over a second floor balcony. One student might be sad at receiving a B grade, while another student in the same class might be thrilled with the B. It has even been shown that activating the facial muscles associated with smiling can induce a state of happiness. All you need to do is hold a pencil across your molars and you can unleash the brain physiology that creates the happiness of pleasure.

Our desire to be happy, while we may not be able to define happiness, has positive and negative effects on our lives and communities. Therefore, it is essential that we understand the complexity of happiness. We need to know the difference between what promotes genuine happiness and why the pursuit of pleasure-based happiness often leads to misery and despair.

The negative aspect of happiness has led insightful thinkers like M. Scott Peck, MD to conclude that "Life is difficult."[2] In fact, Dr. Peck begins his book, *The Road Less Traveled*, with those sobering words. Dr. Peck then goes on to address topics such as Delaying Gratification, The Healthiness of Depression, Escaping from Freedom, and Dedication to Reality. Dr. Peck's topics are not associated with our common experience of happiness as they demand discipline and require us to embrace the discomfort that is often experienced with making the choices that require delaying or deliberately rejecting pleasure-based happiness. However, given our culture's obesity trends, deficit trends, tendency toward hoarding, and accelerating use of anti-anxiety and antidepressant medications, Dr. Peck's arguments might seem, well, un-American.

At this writing, our national debt is currently over 16 trillion dollars ($16,000,000,000,000), it grows by more than 3.88 billion a day, and is expected to exceed 20 trillion dollars in the near future.[3] Meanwhile, several recent studies show that our waistlines are growing every bit as fast, if not faster, than our debt. Obesity rates are projected to rise to over 50% in 39 states by 2030 increasing our already bulging healthcare costs by over 550 billion dollars.[4] Not a happy picture.

The only thing growing faster than our happy-driven debt and waistlines might be the self-storage industry. This is where we stash a lot of purchases we "had to have to be happy." We rarely if ever use these things, many of these stored possessions have little if any value, and most will never see the light of day. There's something eerie and just a bit discomforting about the popular television shows *Storage Wars* and *Hoarders*. Our cluttered living spaces and knick-knack filled cubicles lay bare our happy-driven packrat impulse.

The self-storage industry, for decades, has grown faster than any other segment in the commercial real estate area. Amassing revenues of over 23 billion dollars in 2006 alone.[5] Recent figures show that the total market capitalization of the self-storage industry in the United States is 220 billion dollars. With over 2.21 billion square feet of self-storage in the United States, there is more than 7.3 square feet of storage per U.S. citizen.[6] That means that, even with our expanding waistlines, there is currently enough self-storage space for every American to stretch out in a lounge chair next to a mini fridge stuffed with soda and junk food and still have room for several dust catcher items we have long forgotten. Given the cost of self-storage, there are literally millions of now worthless $20 items which, based on storage costs, cost the self-storer hundreds of dollars each. Not a happy picture.

How do we deal with these impending catastrophes? We self-medicate with a whole host of sugarcoated symptom-suppressing activities. We follow the happiness advice given on pharmaceutical commercials. We run to the corner of happy and healthy to pick-up some cigarettes, cupcakes, candy, ice-cream, prescription drugs, over-the-counter drugs, and pornography. We schedule a national average 7-12 minute first office visit to a conventional doctor and receive a happiness pill or receive some other symptom-masking or suppressing treatment. We buy a book about how to tap into the universe's happy energy source. Again, not a happy picture.

We didn't arrive at our crisis destinations by delaying gratification or dedicating ourselves to reality. However, if we don't shift course quickly, we will all become intimately acquainted with the healthiness of depression and will escape whatever freedom we enjoy in the constraints of morbidity and mortality much sooner than we could have ever imagined. We need to make some super-size changes and we need to start making them now. If we don't see our Pleasure Island donkey ears and tail in the mirror, we're living in denial.

The more we think about our nation's happy meal habits, credit card debt, and psychiatric medications, the more miserable we become. Meanwhile, the only thing our politicians seem to be able to agree on is what donut shop or wine bar they'll meet at to draw new lines in the sand or identify new sources of special interest money. Political happiness has become a game of grandstanding and hoarding special interest campaign money while our country goes to hell in a handbasket.

Our current state of miserable happiness is radically different from the nation our forefathers founded on the bedrock of genuine happiness. When we think about the sacrifices our founders made to gain independence and frame a society based on reasonable and responsible relationships the more alien our consumerist driven, miserable-happy, society looks. Our founding patriots were willing to endure the loss of thousands of lives for over eight horrific Revolutionary War years knowing that the pursuit of happiness was about making personal sacrifices, on a daily basis, for the greater good.

The demand for liberty must have reinforced the idea of personal sacrifice for the common good because the idea seems to have carried over to drafting the Constitution. The Constitution is a document of compromise created by sacrificing personal and provincial interest for the common good. Under those circumstances it is not surprising that the Constitution does not mention I, me, us, or them, but enshrines the notion of "we" and "general welfare" by beginning with the following words: *We the People of the United States, in order to form a more perfect Union, establish justice, insure domestic tranquility, provide for the common defense, promote the general welfare, and secure the Blessings of Liberty to ourselves and our Posterity, do ordain and establish this Constitution for the United States of America.*

Sacrifice and compromise for the general welfare, now that's something to be happy about without feeling miserable. In fact, personal sacrifice and compromise are the stuff of marriage and parenting, community building, and nation strengthening. Sacrifice for the common good is not only the heart and soul of long-term sustainable relationships, it is the heart and soul of our DNA. Sacrifice for the common good is the difference between being connected and being alienated. Personal sacrifice for the general welfare, while uncomfortable and at times painful, is, indeed, what our unalienable right to pursue happiness means.

What is it about our demand for happiness that has moved us so far away from our founding ideals and experiences? That has put us in jeopardy of collapsing under our own weight? Why do we tolerate unhealthy processed and genetically modified food products, national deficits, and a medical system that is certain to create miserable superbugs, financial, and environmental consequences for our children and our grandchildren? Why do we attempt to hoard and store happiness rather than share it and give it away?

Is there an answer to our miserable-happy Pleasure Island dilemma? Can a solution be found? It is precisely these questions that will be addressed and answered below with simple, easy, and completely natural solutions to the mushrooming threats that call into question our children's very survival. It will show that we not only possess the solution, but we've known about the solution from the dawn of human existence. We will show readily available patterns of living that create and sustain lives and communities of permanent genuine happiness. We've all experienced these patterns of living. These patterns are the pattern of our DNA. The following story is an example of our natural capacity to create permanent genuine happiness through community service

It was the spring of 2004, I was coaching a little league baseball team. One player on our team was having a horrible year. He rarely got on the base paths. It was our last game and our last at bat. We were playing the best team in the league. We were down by a run, had the bases loaded, and had two outs.

My team, for the first time all season, was not chasing each other behind the dugout or building mounds in the dugout dirt. My players along with the players, coaches, and parents on the opposing team, were all glued to the game. Our player with the season-long slump was up to bat. We were hoping for a miracle. The pitch was delivered and the ball went rocketing out to right center. He nailed it. A line drive into immortality. As the winning run came across the plate every player on our team charged out of the dugout and mobbed their unlikely hero chanting his name over and over. The other team, while disappointed with the loss, was also caught up in the excitement of our player's magical moment.

The win did not matter and was quickly forgotten. What mattered and lives on was our community, the league, all the parents, and all the players did their job. Little league and all other youth activities, which exist because of parents sacrificing their time and resources, connect our kids, parents, friends, and others to their communities. Being reasonably and responsibly connected is what matters in life. It is what gives life meaning and purpose

All the sacrifices made for our league crystallized in what was going on all year: We were connecting. We were a community acting reasonably and responsibly. We were taking care of each other. Together our community created a moment of permanent genuine happiness that springs from our DNA. It was not difficult. There was no prize money and no trophy. No consumer product to hoard or store. We didn't need to take the kids out for a Twinkie and supersize soda after the game. The magic was that there was no magic or mystery at all. All we had to do was act naturally. Through volunteering and community support we created the most profound experience humanity can achieve, we were connected in a moment of permanent genuine happiness.

I ran into the mom of our hero in the summer of 2012. I told her I planned to include the story in a book I was writing and I asked her if she had any concerns. She lit up. She was excited that I remembered the game and told me it had become a recurring theme of many of her son's school assignments and was a story that was told over and over at family gatherings. It was a powerful experience at the time and it will remain a vivid and powerful experience in the future. To this day, I get goose bumps whenever I relive that amazing season and that magical moment.

Moments of permanent genuine happiness are not confined to exciting hero-type events. Moments of permanent genuine happiness occur many times over the course of a day and are found across the entire range of human experience. They are found in sadness, anger, anxiety, fear, failing, joy, success, and the whole range of human experience. When our anger at an injustice moves us to seek and achieve justice, we create permanent genuine happiness for all who are affected by righting a wrong. We are genuinely happy that we have emotions that call us to action, genuinely happy that our actions confirm that our lives have meaning and purpose, and genuinely happy that our actions inspire others. We create moments of permanent genuine happiness whether we stop to tie a child's shoe or save someone from a burning building. We have the potential to create permanent genuine happiness whenever we act in a reasonable and responsible manner.

In fact, my interest in understanding and promoting genuine happiness sprang from a period of my life where I felt alienated and sought to suppress and mask the pain and discomfort of my alienation with junk food, alcohol, drugs, and a wide range of other unreasonable and irresponsible activities. However, the choices I made only deepened my alienation and left me in many periods of agonizing despair.

I can't deny that I made many years of my life difficult. But, I'm not convinced it had to be that way, or should even be framed in that manner. In fact, as I reflect on the often-desolate path I wandered for decades, I notice that it was always dotted with many moments of genuine happiness.

Hope, like bright yellow dandelion flowers towering above their lush green leaves, would emerge from the smallest cracks in the barren concrete landscape I had created. Those dandelions of hope seemed so smug in knowing that, no matter how hard I'd try, I could not yank them out by the roots. To add insult to resentment, they were ever ready to cast their seeds to the wind and multiply. The persistent messengers of hope that relentlessly appeared in my life confirmed that more than an abundance of dumb luck was keeping me a razor-edge distance from the point of no return.

I eventually found the strength to reach out to others and began to experience a happiness that is only available through reasonable and responsible relationships with myself, others, the planet, and the totality of the universe. I discovered that genuine happiness is not something you seek; it appears when our actions align with our biological demand for reasonable and responsible activity.

Having survived a life with many nightmarish moments, I realize the darkness was permeated with hundreds if not thousands of beautiful, resilient, and persistent dandelions, individuals who had, for no reason, littered my life with random acts of kindness. They were at times painful symptoms of a world full of meaning and purpose that I had tried to mask and suppress with the happiness poison of immediate gratification.

With a healthy family life and master's degrees in comparative religions and clinical psychology, in addition to a doctorate in clinical psychology, I knew I was on solid ground, and I pushed myself to seek answers to the nature of genuine happiness.

I questioned the meaning and purpose of life. Why does humanity suffer through so many unnecessary hardships? Why do we inflict so much damage on our health and the very earth that grants and sustains our lives? Why do we over spend and over consume? What is genuine happiness? Is there even such a thing as genuine happiness? If there is, what is it? Where does it come from? What purpose does it serve?

I had hoped to find answers to these questions from theology; however, while I found clues, I'd run into the concrete walls of religious dogma reinforced by the steel rebar of financial interest. Instead, I turned to behavioral health, the discipline formerly known as psychology to gain entry into the profit-centric, evidence-based conventional medical (EBCM) system monopoly. Psychology changed its name to behavioral health and now, like conventional medicine, pays lip service to our mental and spiritual properties while limiting its treatments to the statistical world of observable data.

Religion and EBCM both are plagued by the very same underlying flaw: dogma. Religious dogma precludes honest questioning for fear of undermining the faith while the dogma of evidence-based research places profits over genuine human science and body-mind-spirit health.

EBCM is truly miraculous. EBCM, grounded in evidence-based dogma, rakes in close to 20% of our gross domestic product, yet is the leading cause of both death and personal bankruptcies in the United States and plays a significant role in destroying our environment. A whopping 42% of Americans currently carry conventional medicine debt and the medical debt they carry is 50% of their overall debt. If they could use the money they pay to conventional medicine to pay off the remainder of their debt they would be debt free. The scientific model that conventional medicine has embraced is called the pragmatic paradigm. The pragmatic paradigm eliminates our mind-spirit properties from research consideration while reducing our body to its observable material elements. Moreover, the EBCM model, while based on the dogma that its research methodology discovers facts, acknowledges that humans cannot know facts—that all human knowledge is imperfect and subject to change. No wonder the pill you take today might be recalled tomorrow after profits have been hoarded and stored and you and your loved ones are in debt, bankrupt, injured or dead. EBCM and its second-class citizen, evidence-based behavioral health, provide no help in learning anything about genuine happiness. The miserable and fatal flaw of EBCM will be discussed in Chapter 4 below.

Before providing an overview of EBCM's pragmatic paradigm and existing options, Chapter 2 will provide a brief history of humanity's search for happiness.

Chapter 2

the history of happiness:
from pleasure to misery and despair

Happiness and moral duty are inseparably connected.
—George Washington

religion and philosophy

Throughout human history, happiness has been viewed as an emotional state characterized by pleasant emotions; in short, happiness has been, in virtually all circumstances, tied to the experience of pleasure. Religious thinkers and philosophers have claimed that the attainment of happiness is our ultimate meaning and purpose and believe is central to the make-up of our spiritual essence and God. According to most world religions, we can only experience the essence of happiness through our relationships to God or only in the presence of God: That is we can only experience the fullness of happiness in the afterlife.

For example, Thomas Aquinas believed that happiness could only be realized as the "Beatific Vision of God's essence in the next life."[7] Islam's absolutes about happiness are similar. Ayed Al-Qarni, in explaining Islam's "Keys to Happiness," claims, "All forms of happiness attained without a firm belief in God, the Almighty are mere illusions."[8]

Buddhist teaching has a slightly different take on happiness. Focused on human experience, Buddhism holds that happiness is ultimately freedom from suffering and contends that suffering is caused by our cravings or desires. Consequently, happiness can only be realized by our ability to overcome cravings of all kinds. First on the list of cravings must be our craving for happiness, as happiness is the impulse for virtually any other cravings. So, oddly enough, it seems that in Buddhism the best way to experience happiness is to reject any desire for happiness.

Philosophers generally believe happiness comes from some conceivable (but not entirely comprehensible) spark, divine or natural, that is guided by our ability to reason. Socrates, for example, sought to live in accordance with his inner impulse for truth (a product of reason), and urged others to find their own way to truth as a path to happiness. Aristotle felt that happiness came when a person fulfilled common and virtuous ends in accordance with reason. Thomas Aquinas believed that, while perfect happiness can only be realized in the afterlife, our earthly experience of happiness is based on our ability to use our practical intelligence in directing our activities. Plato believed our inner spark was manifested in our soul, which allows for happiness when the soul's three dimensions (reason, will, and desire) are in balance. Mencius, a Confucian thinker, felt that happiness could be realized by nourishing our vital force through the practice of virtuous activities, without which our vital force would shrivel away. The holy grail of understanding happiness, then, is to identify what exactly constitutes our "inner spark" soul, vital force, or other descriptive account of our vital force which appears to be restrained by reason. However, as history shows, identifying this inner spark has been easier said than done.

Jonathan Haidt, in his *The Happiness Hypothesis* captures the weight of many religious-philosophical beliefs about happiness in suggesting that "if we rely on balanced wisdom—old and new—eastern and western, liberal and conservative—we can choose directions in our life that lead to satisfaction, happiness and a sense of purpose."[9]

If only it were so easy. Haidt's suggestion makes perfect sense until the opposing and irreconcilable absolutes of the old and new, east and west, liberal and conservative begin to bump heads. In reality, without the bedrock of an absolute on which to drop anchor, compromised solutions end up minimizing the core elements, meaning, and purpose of every human belief system. Such diluted and uncommitted formulas not only leave us in a world without absolutes, they diminish the substance, commitment, and passion of our beliefs and ultimately leave us at the mercy of relativistic manipulation. In short, religious accounts of human happiness, based on speculative belief systems, do not, and cannot, provide a definitive understanding of human meaning, purpose, or genuine happiness.

Thus, while there is some common ground between religious thinkers and philosophers about the nature of happiness, on a whole, it remains a fuzzy concept. Happiness is either tied to God, who we can't comprehend and thus we can't comprehend happiness, or happiness is tied to a mysterious inner spark, soul, vital force, or some other descriptive and speculative "thing" we can't grasp or explain. We are left to muddle along in ignorance, wishful thinking, and hope for some miracle to explain the good, the bad, and the ugly.

behavioral health

Behavioral Health and the human sciences are relatively new participants in the effort to understand and define human happiness. Over the past few decades our understanding of DNA, neurochemicals, genes, and other physiological elements have been correlated with the experience of pleasure, which has become synonymous with happiness. Meanwhile, there has been an intense effort to identify activities that might shed light on behavioral happiness.

In 2002, Martin Seligman[10] summarized the following behavioral findings in respect to the experience of happiness:

1. Pleasure (tasty foods, warm baths, etc.)
2. Engagement (the absorption of an enjoyable activity)
3. Relationships (social ties)
4. Meaning (a perceived quest or belonging to something bigger)
5. Accomplishments (realization of tangible goals)

While all the above items square with our general sense of happiness, they can also be correlated with unhealthy and destructive patterns of living known to result in misery and despair. For example, items 2–5 are all present in terrorist and racist organizations. Item 1 includes unhealthy (albeit tasty) foods that have led to enormous personal and social misery and despair. In fact, in their article, "Sugar and Fat Bingeing Have Notable Differences in Addictive-like Behavior," authors Nicole M. Avena, Pedro Rada, and Bartley G. Hoebel[11] found that sweet taste buds may be largely responsible for producing addictive-like behaviors.

Our pursuit of happiness often results in activities that become habits, which are destructive and leave us in a state of utter despair and misery. In fact, virtually any human tragedy can trace its roots to a pursuit of Pleasure Island happiness. The next chapter will identify the natural consequences of negative and genuine happiness.

Over the course of human history the impact of the pursuit of Pleasure Island happiness has been a root cause of human tragedies, suffering, and misery. The known consequences of pursuing Pleasure Island happiness has resulted in blunt warnings and prohibitions against pleasure seeking. The Ten Commandments are an example of prohibitions against activities carried out in the pursuit of Pleasure Island happiness. The seven deadly sins, shown below, are warnings that the human impulse to experience Pleasure Island-based happiness leads to certain misery.

1. Pride: The desire to be more important than others.
2. Envy: The insatiable desire for something that belongs to another.
3. Greed: An excessive desire for material possessions and wealth.
4. Gluttony: Uncontrolled indulgence.
5. Lust: An intense desire for another person.
6. Sloth: Failure to engage in productive activities.
7. Wrath: Anger that morphs into revenge or spite.

Why do we engage in seven deadly sins activities? We do so because we think such activities and pursuits will make us happy. What is the predictable outcome of participation in seven deadly sins activities? Self and social alienation, disease, soaring unsustainable healthcare costs, debt, health and economic destruction, loss of truthfulness and trust, unsustainable relationships, and ultimately despair and misery. Clearly, while the observable and measurable physiology of happiness falls into a set range, the psychological and spiritual consequences of that physiology are boundless and can lead to the most heinous acts imaginable.

the twinkie dilemma

The Twinkie Dilemma is the choice between pursuing Pleasure Island happiness or embracing the discomfort of doing what we know is reasonable and responsible. We either choose the Twinkie or we reject the Twinkie. It is our choice. If we succumb to a Twinkie temptation such as Seligman's tasty food marker of happiness, we experience the physiology correlated with Pleasure Island happiness. In fact, the mere vision of eating a Twinkie can unleash a physiological sequence that correlates with the feeling of Pleasure Island happiness. However, when we choose to eat the Twinkie we disrupt and impair the healthy functioning of our body-mind-spirit. The disruption of our body-mind-spirit can be so subtle that it can go unnoticed at the level of physiological observation or consciousness. Moreover, we can become so accustomed to an unhealthy state that we believe our unhealthy state is perfect health. However, on the cellular level, just the sugar in a Twinkie (not to mention all the additional chemicals) can contribute a number of serious and harmful health conditions that affect virtually every area of our health. Sugar does not contain any nutritional elements such as minerals, vitamins, or fiber. Moreover, sugar is known to contribute to a wide range of poor health issues including, but not limited to, a destructive effect on the endocrine system, promotion of cancer, and degenerative disease. The same can be said for virtually any other addictive substance or unreasonable activity. Brain chemistry can be significantly changed impairing the natural functioning of our consciousness and our ability to function in a reasonable and responsible manner.

But it doesn't end there.

When we "eat the Twinkie" we can suffer feelings of guilt, remorse, self-doubt, and self-alienation. These mental experiences make us feel unhappy and often increase our craving for more Twinkies to mask or suppress our discomfort. A negative self-perception or self-alienation is reinforced as our waistlines expand and our health deteriorates. The vicious cycle of self-alienation is set in motion by our choice to eat the Twinkie in pursuit of a moment on Pleasure Island. The result is the misery and despair of physical and mental health disease. Moreover, whenever we think about or recall our Twinkie experience our negative self-image is reinforced and we move toward the alienation pole of the wellness continuum. Our self-alienation, at various levels, affects our relationships with others. Whether we admit it or not, the Twinkie has had a negative impact on our body-mind.

But, it doesn't end there.

The choice to eat the Twinkie also has an impact on our spirituality. Our spiritual property, as will be detailed in Chapter 6, is the dimension of our mind that relentlessly pursues and enables us to act reasonably and responsibly. Suffice to say, there is absolutely no circumstance in which eating the Twinkie can be considered reasonable and responsible. Consequently, any and all of our Twinkie moments negatively affect our spirituality.

Altogether, the seemingly harmless act of seeking a moment of Pleasure Island happiness by eating the tasty Twinkie has taken a toll on all core areas of our functioning. Moreover, it may have begun or reinforced a pattern that will lead to miserable consequences. We can develop patterns that lead to obesity, substance abuse, self-alienation, and social alienation, which, in turn, lead to illness, economic hardship, despair, and premature death. Additionally, every time we recall our fateful Twinkie moment, we feel some level of discomfort. Our moment of Twinkie happiness has created a permanent experience of being miserably-happy.

rejecting the twinkie
Eliminating "Twinkie-" caused disease and "Twinkie" healthcare treatments that suppress and mask discomfort rather that address the underlying cause of illness can occur in basically two ways.

The first is to make lifestyle illness uninsurable. Health insurance, like every other type of insurance, should be for accidents and acts of God. Lifestyle illness, which accounts for 90% of illness, is not an accident. Lifestyle illness is a deliberate choice. We have to take personal responsibility for making poor choices. If we eat the Twinkie and wash it down with a supersize soda, or rely on Twinkie treatment pills and procedures, we, not our neighbors, need to pay for our supersize conventional medicine bills. It makes no sense that the country should go bankrupt supporting supersize junk food habits and medical practices that enable the indulgence of unhealthy happiness pursuits to be maintained. The profit-centric pharmaceutical companies and conventional medicine system should pay for all healthcare treatments required to manage the side effects of their products and procedures. Making lifestyle illness uninsurable and making those responsible for side effects responsible for the cost of side effects is a reasonable and responsible option for addressing these problems.

More importantly, it would give everyone the opportunity to experience the health and wellness benefits of reasonable and responsible living. If lifestyle illnesses were not insurable we would not have a healthcare crisis, financial crisis, and our environment would not be becoming an evidence-based pharmaceutical and conventional medicine wasteland.

The second option is to replace the EBCM system with currently available medical systems that treat the whole person, body-mind-spirit.

If we could all just reject the Twinkie, we would have to endure brief periods of "denied craving discomfort" but we would experience the genuine and permanent happiness of a connected and healthy body-mind-spirit. By saying no to the Twinkie, we protect our physiological health, we enhance our mental fortitude, and we provide evidence that we can, in fact, live deeply meaningful lives permeated with the spiritual strength to embrace reasonable and responsible living without any need or desire to visit Pleasure Island.

R, a 67-year-old female, is a great example of how powerful and healing body-mind-spirit work can be. R came to us with high blood pressure. She had a long history of hypertension and had refused medications due to the side effects. Her goal was to reduce her blood pressure naturally. Her blood pressure was very high, at 168/104. I advised her to go to the emergency room, but she refused. She was aware of the risks because other doctors had told her the same thing, but she had gone most of her life without medications and had no intention of becoming dependent on them. She eventually agreed to restart her medications if we could not lower her blood pressure within three weeks.

Other symptoms she reported included anxiety, fatigue, hot flashes, nasal congestion, and poor digestion. Her life was stressful and would continue that way for a while due to a family situation. We ran blood tests, which revealed very low vitamin D levels, inflammation, and an electrolyte imbalance.

She started supplements and changed her diet to an anti-inflammatory diet. R returned three weeks later and her blood pressure was 168/90. She was feeling better, but was still very tired. Her blood pressure at home reported averaging 145-165/ 80-85. We continued to work on her energy, recommended a vitamin D replacement, and diet recommendations. She was very compliant and did everything we asked her to do. R returned again three weeks later and her blood pressure was 158/82. She reported feeling incredible, better than she had felt in years! She reported decreased anxiety, sleep was more restful, and she had more energy. Her hot flashes were greatly reduced and her bowel movements were much better. We continue to monitor her blood pressure and it is expected to keep coming down.

R was willing to do whatever it took to get her health back. She reports that not only is she safer with lowered blood pressure, but is also a much happier person and is coping with the stress better. When we have health, we can deal with the stress of life easier! This is an example of what we can achieve if we are willing to do what is reasonable and responsible to work with our body-mind-spirit.

The outcome of each Twinkie challenge has a lasting effect. Recall something you accomplished by denying a comfort craving. It can be anything: Completing a difficult task, exercising, disclosing an error, oversight, apologizing for a wrong, or choosing an organic apple instead of a piece of sugar-drenched apple pie. How did you feel then? And how do you feel about your reasonable and responsible action now? A frequent response is that such acts, while involving some discomfort or denied gratification, make us happy in a special and empowering way. We experience the humble yet powerful happiness of caring for ourselves and others in need. We know we nourished our body and fortified our mental-spiritual capacity to act reasonably and responsibly. Moreover, we realize that such experiences of happiness can remain so vivid that years later they still bring a smile to our face and peace to our heart and soul.

Genuine permanent happiness is an unintended consequence of reasonable and responsible activity. The experience of genuine happiness is rarely expected and in many situations seems to come out of nowhere. Yet, while it might seem to come from some unexplained universal source of happiness, it, in fact, comes from within us. It comes from living within ourselves. It comes from our deliberate effort to do what we know is the reasonable and responsible thing to do moment-to-moment. It comes from the wisdom of our body-mind-spirit and our choice to defend the integrity of our body-mind-spirit by acting in accordance with the demands of our body-mind-spirit. In 12-step programs serenity comes from doing the reasonable and responsible irrespective of the discomfort experienced.

We face Twinkie Dilemma challenges many times over the course of a day. These challenges are the subplot of every human story. The story of Pinocchio is a classic example. The more Pinocchio pursued pleasure the more alienated he became from his dream of becoming human. In the end, Pinocchio's Pleasure Island life was turning him into a miserable jackass.

Pinocchio's Pleasure Island is our destiny when we confuse the unreasonable and irresponsible pursuit of pleasure with genuine happiness by mindlessly popping a pill every time we catch a cold or have a fever, consume junk food, substance abuse, or engage in any other body-mind-spirit numbing "happy" activity in hopes of experiencing some Pleasure Island happiness.

So what exactly is our body-mind-spirit and how do we know if an activity supports or harms our body-mind-spirit?

As discussed above, theology while claiming that happiness is tied to God, also claims that we can never fully comprehend God, which means we can never fully comprehend happiness. Thus, religious dogma, doctrine, and ordinary teaching can only offer a conceivable, but not comprehensible explanation of body-mind-spirit health. In fact, reliance on religious dogma and doctrine can be dangerous. In the absence of an explanation of our body-mind-spirit health that is both conceivable and comprehensible, religions, which all emerged from reasonable and responsible insights about human meaning and purpose, are easily distorted and frequently used to pursue the seven deadly sins, and religious conflicts have and continue to inflict a horrific level of suffering across the globe. It should be clear that through the centuries, in the present, and in the predictable future, religious manipulation has been and will continue to be, a significant source of human suffering and misery.

evidence-based conventional medicine:
the pornographic approach to health and happiness

In contrast to theology's absolutes about the incomprehensible, Evidence-Based Conventional Medicine (EBCM) claims all human science must be based on observable data. Thus to achieve happiness humans must be reduced to their observable material properties and the behavior that material properties prescribe. We go to a conventional doctor or behavioral health center when our unreasonable and irresponsible lifestyle renders us unhappy. We are given material-only drugs or behavioral advice that masks or suppresses the natural consequence of our unreasonable and irresponsible lifestyle so we can continue our life on Pleasure Island while wearing our chemical-colored glasses. However, humans are more than the sum of our observable material properties and behavior. EBCM, in rejecting our mental-spiritual properties from its evidence-based model of science, disqualifies itself as science. Science demands a comprehensive and systematic explanation. Comprehensive explanation must include all available data. Thus in the case of human science the data must include both the observable data of our material properties and behavior and the non-observable data of our mind-spirit properties. It is only by including both our material and mental properties of our body-mind-spirit that we can develop a comprehensive and systematic human science. By excluding our mind-spirit properties from its research model EBCM is similar to pornography. Both pornography and EBCM only concern themselves with the physical properties of humanity. The profits gained from a purely physical approach are as mind-blowing as its destructive impact.

The material-only data of EBCM is not comprehensive and therefore can't be systematic. By eliminating our mental-spiritual properties EBCM research has little if anything to do with the reality of what a human is. EBCM, by applying statistics to its material-only data is in fact not science, but merely statistics masquerading as science. In fact, not one single finding of EBCM is acknowledged to be a fact. That is, there is not one finding of EBCM that is not subject to revision. To wit, after the approved pill or procedure kills and harms thousands, the recalled approved pill and now prohibited procedure is simply another member of evidence-based conventional medicine's ever-expanding list of killers.

In the absence of legitimate body-mind-spirit science is it not surprising that EBCM, like religious dogma and doctrine, is easily distorted and used to pursue the seven deadly sins—aside from pride. The EBCM claim that, "We're the best medical system in the world with the best doctors." Not 37th best, and dropping, according to the World Health Organization! First and foremost is greed. Make no mistake about it, EBCM is about money and monopoly.

Obviously then, what is needed is a body-mind-spirit-based science that can hold the EBCM profiteers accountable. With such a science we can confidently determine if the happiness experienced by eating a Twinkie is good or bad. Such an understanding will not only integrate the seemingly irreconcilable views of science and theology, it will provide us with an absolute definition of genuine happiness and the role it plays in human meaning and purpose.

Emergent Property Theory, presented in Chapter 5, identifies just such a genuine science-based model. It is impossible to overstate the importance of this groundbreaking body-mind-spirit model of human science. It is a game changing understanding of the meaning and purpose of human life. However, it involves some technical information. Nonetheless, gaining a basic understanding of the concepts of Emergent Property Theory is critical to understanding both body-mind-spirit health and genuine happiness.

However, prior to presenting the chapter on Emergent Property Theory we will provide an overview of the gaps and inconsistencies of the EBCM system.

Given that our health and wellness are of paramount importance to our genuine happiness, the next section of the book will review how and why EBCM is not science, and why, in addition to the economic and environmental damage EBCM causes, EBCM causes more health problems than it solves. In fact, it will be shown that evidence-based research and treatments, based on discredited dogma of logical positivism as a human science methodology, are not science-based treatments at all.

Lacking a scientific foundation, EBCM has morphed into a profit-centric Whack-A-Mole healthcare system that claims to increase our happiness by whacking the discomforting symptoms of our body-mind-spirit with mallet blows made up of pills, procedures, and devices. However, as we all are becoming miserably aware, our whacked body-mind-spirit symptom moles whack back. Unfortunately, we, not the profit-centric whackers, pay the price of the whack-back pill and procedure moles. The EBCM whackers only make more profits by providing more mole-whacking pills and procedures as we are pushed down the path of whacking side effects with more pills and more procedures.

EBCM dogma, referred to as the pragmatic paradigm, is based on a contradictory combination of logical positivism and representational theory. Logical positivism claims that evidence-based science can produce facts while representational theory claims that there is no possibility of producing a fact. Evidence-based proponents acknowledge the fact that there are no facts and thus, acknowledge that all of their research findings and treatments may cause great harm. The harm is made abundantly apparent by FDA adverse reactions recalls due to side effects caused by the evidence-based treatments used in EBCM practice. Adverse reactions have killed millions and permanently injured millions more. Knowing the damage done and certain the damage will continue, EBCM profiteers have happily adopted the pragmatic paradigm language. In other words, given that we know, there is no such thing as a fact, EBCM profiteers nonetheless insist the show must go on and the money must flow. It is the pragmatic way to transfer trillions of dollars from the general population to the EBCM system.

Representational theory, also referred to as social constructivism or post-modern philosophy, in contrast to logical positivist based evidence-based research, claims humans can not know facts. According to representational theory, the human biological processes and the cultural/historical filters we rely on to turn sensory data into concepts blurs our understanding of reality. Because of these filters, all research findings and treatments are subject to change or revision. Thus, while EBCM promotes itself as credible science, EBCM must, at the same time, acknowledge that all EBCM research and treatments are built on the shifting sands of its very own pragmatic paradigm. Moreover, given that science is based on a comprehensive and systematic attempt to gain a closer approximation of a research target to its reality, EBCM's exclusive focus on observable material data of physical science does not and can not consider the reality of our non-observable mental properties. In other words, EBCM is not comprehensive and, therefore, has no possibility of approximating the reality of what a human is.

EBCM profiteers have a field day manipulating evidence-based research to have evidence-based products approved by the evidence-based Food and Drug Administration. The game is to use statistics to show that the product or procedure, worth billions of dollars, will cause less discomfort and disease than the symptoms the billion dollar product is designed to whack. The profiteers are not only brilliant at their craft, they also control all elements of the EBCM system.

The EBCM system created a crisis in which all evidence-based researchers, educators, and healthcare providers must defend their professional practices while acknowledging they do not know if their activities are more helpful or more harmful. Thus, while they do know that virtually all EBCM treatments have harmful side effects that can cause permanent damage and often death as stated in virtually every one of their happy people advertisements, they drink the evidence-based Kool-Aid while ignoring the personal bankruptcies, national debt, and environmental damage their pragmatism causes.

It is a pragmatism that has reduced EBCM to a field of smoke and mirror statistical manipulation governed by profit potential. EBCM has turned medical science into a roulette wheel. Whether consumers win or lose, the house makes a profit. Lonergan captures the underlying deception of evidence-based human science when he points out:

> *The scandal still continues that men* [and women], *while they tend to agree on scientific questions, tend to disagree in the most outrageous fashion on basic philosophic issues. So they disagree about the activities named knowing about the relation of those activities to reality, and about reality itself.* [12]

The fact that evidence-based "science" is not based on facts exposes major gaps in EBCM's understanding of human functioning, change, development, health, and happiness. It also exposes the fact that EBCM's primary motivation is money and monopoly.

EBCM reality check

As stated above, far from creating genuine happiness, the EBCM system has, is, and will continue to be a leading cause of our health, economic, and environmental misery and despair. Not only does the EBCM system permanently injure millions annually, it is the leading cause of death in the United States.[13] Additionally, it gobbles-up close to 20% of our economy and is the leading cause of personal bankruptcies (62%).[14] It is also creating untreatable superbugs and is destroying our environment.[15] EBCM defines being miserable-happy.

Understanding the dogmatic claims and myths on which EBCM is based and operates will explain why we can find little help in the EBCM system for creating healthy and genuinely happy individuals and communities. In fact, it is our Kool-Aid drinking hope and prayer that the EBCM system will come up with the miracle cure that will create Pleasure Island happiness for us where all illness and even death are eliminated from human experience. We have all become wowed by the miracle of modern medicine and are almost immune from the daily media reports of modern medicine disasters. The following chapter will discuss the underlying flaw of EBCM which has not only caused a steady downpour of EBCM tragedies, but has also created havoc in our economy and is destroying our environment.

Chapter 3

EBCM's fatal flaw

Logical positivists (evidence-based researchers) have never taken psychology into account in their epistemology, but they affirm that logical beings and mathematical beings are nothing but linguistic structures.

—Jean Piaget

The fatal flaw of EBCM is two-fold. On the one hand, EBCM is based on logical positivism. Logical positivism claims all science must be based exclusively on observable data. Thus our mental-spiritual data is considered meaningless because it cannot be observed. There is no mental-spiritual evidence-based research. None. However, it is precisely our mental-spiritual properties are what make us humans and determine our health and genuine happiness.

In the first instance, logical positivism has been systematically and comprehensively discredited as a basis for human science. As stated above, logical positivism demands that all research data, if it is to be scientific, must be observable. Thus, evidence-based research excludes our mental and spiritual experience from science because neither are observable. According to evidence-based research, if research data is not observable it is meaningless. By excluding our unobservable, yet experienced, mental and spiritual data from its research EBCM cannot offer a comprehensive or systematic explanation of anything having to do with human health, wellness, meaning, purpose, or happiness. EBCM stands on an unstable and extremely dangerous one-legged stool of material-only research data.

Secondly, and ironically, it is the human mind, deemed meaningless in EBCM, which created EBCM and is responsible for the existence of every EBCM research study and treatment. There would be no evidence-based study without a human mind. Moreover, it is the reality of our mental properties that utterly destroys any possibility that evidence-based research can form the basis of human science.

The well-meaning logical positivist hope was that a unified science could be developed based on the following evidence-based principles.

1. Scientific method must be the same for all science (physical and human science).
2. The purpose of science must be to comprehensively and systematically explain and predict.
3. Scientific findings must be reliable and verifiable (findings must be factual).
4. Science must avoid common sense bias in research.

5. Science must be judged by logic through the application of deductive reasoning.

6. Experiments must be able to verify a finding of *fact* anytime and anywhere.

However, because humans have minds, the possibility of creating an exclusively evidence-based human science is impossible. In fact, having established the above criterion, the founders of logical positivism almost immediately came to the conclusion that none of the required evidence-based principles applied to human science. The positivist criterion cannot be applied to humans because humans, unlike the material world of rocks and computers, have biologically based body-mind-spirit properties. If the human mind-spirit, is eliminated from evidence-based research, then evidence-based research cannot claim to be science. By eliminating our mind-spirit evidence-based research is not comprehensive. Moreover, anything that is not comprehensive cannot be systematic. If evidence-based research is neither comprehensive nor systematic it cannot be reliable or verifiable.

Additionally, the mind-spirit that evidence-based research arbitrarily eliminates, "science," absolutely discredits its claims that experiments can find facts. To wit, our body-mind-spirit properties, unlike rocks and computers, assign meaning to our world. Meaning assignment is subjective. Climbing a rock is exciting to some and terrifying to others. A robot design to climb a rock, in contrast to a human, assigns no meaning to the experience whatsoever. Thus, verification of all logical positivist requirements was deemed impossible due to the fact that the positivist believed the subjective dimension of human experience eliminates the possibility of verifying a finding of fact anytime, anywhere. In fact, it led the founders of logical positivism to conclude that facts do not exist. Facts are simply subjective interpretations of observable data. According to their own pragmatic paradigm there does not exist a single fact in EBCM research or treatments.

The fact that human knowledge is mediated by biological processes and historical/cultural influences which turn sensory data and abstract mental data into human knowledge utterly destroys the fact-verifying dream of logical positivists. Additionally, quantum physics demonstrates that everything changes moment-to-moment. The list of pragmatic facts that destroys the possibility of ever finding a fact has mushroomed. In fact, A. J. Ayer, considered a founding father of logical positivism, stated "...the most important defect of logical positivism was that *all of it was false* ...the reductionism just doesn't work."[16]

Not to be deterred, evidence-based proponents pushed ahead and sought fame and fortune by exploiting the general public's naïve belief that evidence-based "science" could rid humanity of illness, disease, and virtually any experience of discomfort.

To address the human "mind-spirit-problem" evidence-based positivists have worked tirelessly to construct brain theory models that can eliminate our body-mind-spirit properties by turning our body-mind-spirit properties into material computer-like properties (see Appendix B for an overview of how positivists have attempted to model our body-mind-spirit properties into non-biological computers).

Dennett, a leading positivist proponent, captures both the problem our body-mind-spirit properties impose on evidence-based research and summarizes the EBCM solution to the mind problem in stating:

> *Even if mental events are not among the data of science, this does not mean we cannot study them scientifically... the challenge is to construct a theory of mental events, using the data that scientific method* [evidence-based research] *permits.*[17]

In effect, what evidence-based proponents propose is to change the reality of our body-mind-spirit properties to fit the evidence-based model of science. Thus, as Taylor points out, by constructing a material-only theory of mental events, what positivist proponents generally mean is to construct "a reductive explanation of human action and experience in physiological and ultimately in physical and chemical terms."[18] The mantra of evidence-based proponents appears to be: If reality doesn't fit your profit-generating model of science, then reality, not the profit-generating model, has to change.

As indicated above, the primary method evidence-based proponents use to change our body-mind-spirit into physical and chemical components is by turning them into computer systems. However, computer theories of our body-mind-spirit are not science. Computer theories of our mind-spirit are nothing other than science fiction.

EBCM compounds the problem of excluding our body-mind-spirit properties from "science" by reducing the material matter to the smallest component it can isolate. That is, EBCM is radically reductionist. In fact, reductionism is the only possible option evidence-based research has to treat illness. However, by reducing wholes to material-only component parts, evidence-based research cannot address the fact that wholes are always greater than, and qualitatively different from, the sum of their parts.

Having summarily lopped off our body-mind-spirit properties from the get-go, EBCM then concocts material-only chemical treatments and/or surgical procedures to whack or remove an isolated material component or components of the whole. The problem is that by whacking a component of our body-mind-spirit whole, the whole is whacked and weakened and can be permanently damaged or destroyed.

Limited to observable data the EBCM can only offer Whack-A-Mole-type medicine. EBCM uses the heavy mallets of material-only drugs and surgery to whack isolated material elements of our body-mind-spirit correlated with an EBCM defined symptom of illness or disease. However, the EBCM-defined symptoms are often body-mind-spirit warning signs of unhealthy patterns that need to be understood and addressed with body-mind-spirit treatments, not whacked by chemicals or removed by surgery. By whacking or removing the warning signs of illness, EBCM not only masks or suppresses the warning signs, it disrupts and can destroy our natural healing properties. Side effects caused by EBCM treatments pop up whenever symptoms are whacked by EBCM treatments. The side effects are then whacked, and then, as the whacking process accelerates, our natural wellness and healing properties become overwhelmed and fail. With enough whacking, our increasingly decrepit survival becomes totally dependent on being whacked with more costly pills and surgery.

EBCM, rigidly trapped by its evidence-based dogma, cannot address the health and wellness of our body-mind-spirit. Thus, the positivist dogma of EBCM has become EBCM's fatal flaw.

In the meantime, while the profiteers' advertisements market a continuous stream of profit-centric EBCM miracle claims and cures, our environment becomes overrun with toxic residue, we're forced into personal bankruptcy to pay for our whacking, and our national debt comes closer and closer to default.

A recent Chicago Sun-Times report provides an example of how the system works and how we've become willing Kool-Aid drinkers. The report detailed a scary and happy threatening experience of Chicago Bull basketball star Luol Deng. Deng reported the unhappy and uncomfortable experience of flu-like symptoms. In response his EBCM doctors fearing viral meningitis, recommended an emergency spinal tap (Deng did not have meningitis). That, according to Deng, "is when it all went downhill... I did the spinal tap and after that I just didn't respond well, I started having severe headaches, was struggling to walk. I started feeling really weak. I started throwing up—constant diarrhea. I couldn't control my body—really. Because of that I lost [15 pounds]. And I'm still just trying to get back, just trying to get right. I still don't feel right... It was scary. I've never been through anything like that in my whole life."[19]

Most of us know someone who has had a similar, or worse, EBCM incident. My mom had heartburn. She was rushed to the hospital and the conventional doctors, misdiagnosing a heart attack, gave her nitro; it almost killed her.

What is our response to such experiences? It's often similar to Deng's. Deng returned to the hospital, twice for more whacking. Moreover, at the end of his ordeal Deng, like most of us, reported he was grateful for the experience. He is reported to have stated, "They wanted to make sure I didn't have meningitis. I'm thankful they wanted to make sure."[20] Talk about drinking the Whack-A-Mole Kool-Aid.

It is scary to think how much we have to pay in increased insurance premiums and healthcare profiteer taxes for the cumulative cost of the thousands of EBCM incidents like Deng's that occur on a daily basis. You would think the hospital would have waived any charges and compensated Deng, the Bulls, and Bull fans for their mistake. Not a chance. They probably think Deng's Kool-Aid thank you validates their misdiagnosis and all the costs associated with it. I have news for you, Luol, there's a good chance you'll never be the same. There is a good chance the whacking you received will lead to more whacking down the road. There's a chance you'll be "thanking" EBCM for the thoroughness of their whacking the rest of your life.

EBCM is merely the Twinkie Dilemma on steroids. The broken health and happiness promises made by EBCM's miracle myths are a primary cause of our misery and despair.

Our fear that illness and death will strip us of our happiness has played, and continues to play, a critical role in the creation of the profit-centric EBCM healthcare monopoly. The monopoly is comprised of a wide range of private, government, and EBCM financed non-profit organizations that promoted EBCM dogma while excluding any competing healthcare systems or treatments from gaining access to the United States healthcare delivery system.

Evidence-based dogma defines all aspects of the monopolistic profit-centric EBCM system. Drug and device manufacturers, medical procedure developers, conventional medical schools, private and governmental insurance providers, governmental regulatory agencies, and any other organization that wants to attain full and equal participation in the profit-centric conventional health care system must drink the profit-centric evidence-based Kool-Aid. Web sites for virtually all these organizations explicitly state that those without evidence-based credentials need not apply. Once in, any deviation from the dogma is not tolerated. EBCM is a cynical, deceptive, bullying, and brutal enterprise designed for profits. It is not concerned with health, wellness, our economy, our environment, nor genuine body-mind-spirit wellness. The following section will provide an overview of how the EBCM's powerful profiteers have created an EBCM system that is like an ever-expanding whirlpool, which sucks in virtually every private and governmental healthcare related enterprise. The whirlpool was created by, and is sustained by, the profits hoarded in the profiteers' bank accounts at the bottom of the drain. Presented below are two examples of the EBCM whirlpool in action.

United States Preventive Services Task Force (USPSTF)
USPSTF is an evidence-based organization created in response to the magnitude of deaths and injuries occurring in the conventional medical system. The USPSTF claims to have developed a science grading system in which the evidence-based methodology of EMCM gets an A. However, as stated earlier, evidence-based research methodology is not human science. Evidence-based human science is an ideological

dogma propped-up by statistics. Nonetheless, the USPSTF proclaims evidence-based research methodology to be the gold standard research methodology for human science. This gold standard grading system (which has been revised several times) categorizes science on how research is designed, not on scientific principles or clinical outcomes. In fact, the grading system grades research before it is conducted. Research which adheres to evidence-based (double-blind research) requirements is given an A grade before the research is conducted. The grading system is like paying a contractor $50,000 in advance and giving them an A before anybody shows up at the worksite. The USPSTF, is the first and only institution in human history to grade science.

The USPSTF describes itself as an "…independent, volunteer panel of national experts in prevention and evidence-based medicine."[21] As an independent evidence-based group of evidence-based experts, the USPSTF site provides the following language to encourage a "diversified' group of evidence-based *only* proponents":

To obtain a diversity of evidence-based only perspectives, qualified applicants and nominees must, at a minimum, demonstrate knowledge, expertise, and national leadership in… Implementation of evidence-based recommendations in clinical practice, including at the clinician-patient level, practice level, and health system level.[22]

In short, a diversity of perspectives is encouraged as long as it does not impinge upon the rigidity of evidence-based dogma.

While the EBCM system in the United States is by far the most expensive medical system in the world, it is ranked 37th in effectiveness by the World Health Organization. Improvement in the ranking is currently being sought. The improved ranking is being sought, not by changing the system or addressing EBCM's fatal flaw, but by changing the grading system and other quality measures used by evidence-based profiteers to evaluate evidence-based outcomes. The grading system, based solely on the opinions of evidence-based profiteers, will continue to be tweaked and, if necessary, overhauled, to defend and sustain EBCM's monopoly and profits.

The EBCM system is further supported by the evidence-based United States Food and Drug Administration (FDA).

the FDA: EBCM's whack-a-mole watchdog

Given EBCM's history of unimaginable Whack-A-Mole healthcare disasters, the FDA, an EBCM club member, was compelled to create procedures to track adverse events caused by evidence-based and developed prescription drugs, devices, and procedures. However, given that EBCM profits are in the trillions of dollars, the FDA has become a Whack-A-Mole game itself with a long queue of EBCM entities and profiteer financed consumer groups waiting to swing their lobby mallets in hopes that a big dollar FDA drug approves. In this respect Daniel P. Carpenter states, the "U.S. Food and Drug Administration (FDA) drug review bears a structural similarity to many decisions made by other regulatory agencies: high uncertainty, low reversibility, avoidance of observable error, and high political stakes that induce lobbying by interested parties." [23]

The FDA is pressured to approve miracle treatments, while at the same time it is being charged with monitoring and recalling miracle treatments due to adverse effects. Many lobbied for and approved "miracle" drugs and products are later found to have "serious outcomes [that] include death, hospitalization, disability, congenital anomaly and/or other serious outcomes." [24] The FDA cannot hope to effectively contend with the profit-centric EBCM requests it receives, which all pressure the FDA to save "Johnny's" life by approving their latest miracle cure. Thus, as Paul Leber, an FDA representative, in addressing the safety of pharmaceuticals stated, "Because no pharmacologically active drug substance is entirely free of risk, the conclusion that a drug has been shown to be 'safe for use,' is actually no more than an opinion… Accordingly, 'risks to benefit assessments' are inherently arguable, all the more so because each turns not only on personal sentiments about the nature of risks and benefits of a drug, but upon incomplete and imperfect information concerning the drug's risk."[25] Opinion is not science. It is lobbying driven by potential profits and stock price positioning.

Due to the fatal flaws of EBCM research, The Gold Sheet www.elsevierbi.com, an organization that reviews EBCM recalls, reports the steady climb in recalls averaging over 50% in some years. The Gold Sheet review is conservative in its reports as a huge percentage of deaths and injuries are never reported. Yet we not only drink the Whack-A-Mole EBCM Kool-Aid, we can't imagine being happy without it.

Oddly enough, EBCM rationalizes all the destruction it causes based on the second pillar of its pragmatic paradigm foundation, representational theory. The next section will provide an overview of representational theory and how EBCM uses representational theory to explain why EBCM disasters are to be expected, why our personal and national wealth should be transferred to the EBCM system, why our children's inheritance should be transferred to the EBCM system, why we should go bankrupt paying for healthcare, and why the destruction of our environment and superbugs are unavoidable.

representational theory

Representational theory emerged from the fact that, in addition to our material properties and unlike material-only computer systems, we have biological minds. Our body-mind-spirit consciousness enables us to understand and apply meaning to what we experience. For example, we have all experienced love or loving something. However, while we name our experience "love," the word love can never fully capture our experience of love. The word love is like the tip of an iceberg when it comes to capturing the whole of our experience. Like love, all words are inadequate in capturing the totality of whatever we are attempting to describe. The words we use to describe evidence-based findings are all conditioned by the limits of language and the impact our historical time, culture, and body-mind-spirit biology have on the language we use.

In addition to the fact that language can never capture the totality of what we've experienced and know, experience is strictly the experience of the experiencing individual. No two people have the identical experience of anything. Thus the fact that we have conscious awareness utterly destroys any and all of EBCM miracle cure claims because the mental acts of our conscious awareness, unlike the material matter of physical science, demand that we apply subjective meaning to what we know. Moreover, given that our experience changes moment-to-moment we rarely have the identical experience of anything. For example, coffee might be valued in the morning while avoided right before bedtime. In fact, based on our understanding of quantum physics, we know that the material world is in constant flux.

Representational theorists have identified mental factors in human perception, historical, and cultural factors that they claim reduce factual knowledge to interpretation. In short, representational theorists claim human knowledge is not a process of fact-finding. Human knowledge is, according to representational theory, as McCarthy points out, the process of constructing viewpoints at the "intersection of biology and culture."[26] Additionally, the language we use to express a viewpoint, plays a dominant role in how we objectify and assign meaning to our body-mind-spirit experience that we attempt to capture and convey to others through language.

In this respect, as McCarthy explains, without benefit of language, human knowledge would be restricted to "the immediate perceptual intuition of sensible objects."[27] In other words, without language our knowledge would be limited to observable data only. However, based on our ability to use the abstract symbolism of language, our ability to understand the world around us is dramatically increased. Through language, we cannot only express what we experience through sensory data, we can express what we can imagine. Thus, as McCarthy states, "the [positivist] model of the directly intuited world (observable sensory data) has given way to the ampler world mediated by symbolic expression."[28] Symbolic expression is not a material reality. Symbolic expression is the product of our biological body-mind-spirit properties.

Symbolic expression, a core aspect of human knowledge, is made possible by our body-mind-spirit properties and is expressed through language or some other symbolic expression like art. Therefore, the EBCM claim that human knowledge consists of objectified sensory facts cannot explain the symbolic dimension of human knowledge. Our biological processes, according to representational theory, turn sensory data into mental pictures and the language we use to express those pictures filters and creates gaps between our understanding of the objects and the objects themselves.

In representational theory, then, the only absolute is the claim that all human knowledge is constructed representations of our experience rather than logically reduced facts. What we know is our body-mind-spirit interpretation of the object and event we attend to. Given that human knowledge is interpretation and not fact, logical positivism's verification criterion went out the window.

The common thread in representational dogma is, as Messer & Wachtel point out, that there "is no possibility of uncovering general principles, laws, or truths about human nature."[29] Accordingly,

Richardson, et. al., (1999) argue that representational theorists have come to the conclusion that "it is time to bite the bullet and acknowledge the fundamental truth (any irony intended) that all our beliefs and values are strictly relative."[30]

Representational theory has identified several factors that inform the manner in which we interpret, rather than develop factual knowledge about our experience, and apply meaning to our world. Those factors created what philosophers referred to "the problem of the bridge." The result of this confrontation between us and the objects and events we encounter creates a bridge or gap between reality as it is and our perception and interpretation of reality. Moreover, given that everything changes moment-to-moment, any perception and interpretation we construct can only apply to the object being understood at the moment of our experiencing and interpreting.

Representational theory has had a dramatic impact on the human sciences. It has resulted in the current human science field acceptance of its status as quasi-science. Recognizing that evidence-based human science is incapable of producing scientific facts, the EBCM profiteers decided they could, nonetheless, construct an evidence-based goose that could lay golden eggs. Moreover, they discovered that representational theory, far from impeding their progress, could be used to explain away the disasters their golden egg deceptions have and will continue to produce.

gaps in representational theory

Representational theory claims that human knowledge is not factual knowledge. Human knowledge is always biased by the filters that separate the knower from the would-be known object or event. However, the story of our filters is incomplete. Yes, biological, linguistic, and cultural factors filter the objects and experience we attend to, however, what the representational theorists have neglected to do is identify the very structure from which our mental filters arise. The source of the filters is the human body-mind-spirit. Thus, as McCarthy points out, "representational theorists have regularly neglected to trace these truth-bearing intentional signs, logical or linguistic, to their source in the intentional subject."[31] That is, what the human mind evidence-based positivist and the EBCM profiteers claim, is not open to scientific research and in all likelihood does not exist.

In the absence of identifying how mental representations are created, conserved, and refined in our body-mind-spirit properties, representational theory cannot offer a comprehensive and systematic explanation of what human knowledge is. Identifying and locating the source of our mental representation in human consciousness which emerges from our body-mind-spirit is a fundamental departure in our understanding of our body-mind-spirit and our understanding of what human knowing is. It is, as will be argued in Chapter 6, an understanding of human knowing and knowledge that is not subject to further change. It is an absolute. The structure and operations of human consciousness overcomes the problem of the bridge exposed by representational theory and provides the basis for creating a comprehensive and systematic body-mind-spirit science. That is, a genuine human science.

Like the behaviorist who focuses on observable behavior rather than our body-mind-spirit properties and processes that produce the behavior, representational theorists have focused on the observable products of perception and interpretation or the material properties of our sensory systems rather than the sum of those parts which is our consciousness. Recognizing consciousness as the agent of our body-mind-spirit properties and processes allow us to overcome representational theory's oversights and logical positivism's mono-material limitations.

Representational theory's impact on EBCM has dramatically expanded in the past several decades. In fact, EBCM hedges all its cure claims on representational arguments. EBCM's reliance on representational theory is a critical element in EBCM strategy for defending the catastrophic damage it causes to our health, financial system, and environment. The representational foundation of EBCM is why EBCM medicine dogma is referred to as the pragmatic paradigm. Knowing that all EBCM research and treatments are subject to change (i.e., FDA adverse reaction recalls). EBCM confidently boasts that in all cases, good, bad, and ugly, they put their best foot forward based on the limitations of "gold standard" evidence-based science. In playing the pragmatic card EBCM claims its treatments are "state-of-the-art" and that while there is always a significant probability of damage, permanent damage, or death, it's better than doing nothing. After all, there are no profits to be made sitting on your hands and not making money on state-of-the-art treatments irrespective of the outcome. Death and destruction are simply collateral damage inherent to profit-centric pragmatism.

EBCM's acknowledgement that its representational foundation undercuts all its health and happiness claims is little more than lip service. The representational foundation of the EBCM paradigm only makes a cameo appearance in the form of a "we're not perfect" shoulder shrug in response to the daily reports of EBCM disasters.

Representational theory's insistence that all human understanding is relative is a perfect fit for EBCM's shift from a foundationless science to the foundationless statistical construct of evidence-based research masquerading as human science. The probability and chance of statistics in many respects mimic the claim of representational theory. Both provide a pragmatic "we're doing the best we can do given our inability to know anything" excuse for virtually any catastrophe EBCM causes and both provide a license to reap huge profits while spinning the roulette wheel with our health, wellness, and genuine happiness.

Summary: EBCM's destructive impact on our health and happiness should not be news to anyone. There is a daily downpour of articles, books, and media documents that report EBCM's debilitating health, economic, and environmental catastrophes. As stated above, we spend close to 20% of our gross national product on EBCM and EBCM is the leading cause of death and permanent injuries in the United States. EBCM also creates untreatable superbugs, causes unsustainable national debt, and accounts for over 62% of personal bankruptcies. Among many other significant problems, EBCM is also causing massive damage to our aquatic life and environment. Nonetheless, we drink the EBCM Kool-Aid myths and believe our happiness will certainly one day depend on an EBCM miracle cure.

Our acceptance of the EBCM system is driven by our fear that illness and death will strip us and our loved ones of happiness. EBCM markets its pills, products, and procedures based on our fears. The abysmal impact EBCM has on our health, economy, and environment is suppressed and masked by misleading advertisements, media campaigns, lobbying, and misinformation campaigns about non-EBCM professions. However, our unquestioned deification of EBCM as a God-like protector of our health and happiness is relentlessly moving us toward the alienation pole of the alienation-connectedness continuum of wellness and is the leading cause of our misery and despair.

EBCM's fatal flaw is that it is based on dogma, not science. The principle dogma of EBCM is that all science must be based on observable data and observable data alone. However, human health, wellness, and genuine happiness have little to do with the observable properties of material matter or observable behavior. It is the unobservable properties of our body-mind-spirit that determine our health, wellness, and genuine happiness. In fact, the observable material properties of biology can only be separated from our biological body-mind-spirit by death. EBCM's response to our body-mind-spirit properties is to claim they are illusionary and can be eliminated by reducing our body-mind-spirit to observable material matter. By eliminating our body-mind-spirit properties from its research model EBCM has turned the balanced three-legged stool of our body-mind-spirit into EBCM's one-legged daredevil act.

There is no evidence-based research or evidence-based treatments that can consider the impact our consciousness, as an emergent property of our body-mind-spirit, has on our health, wellness, or genuine happiness. EBCM claims of treating our mind-spirit properties are marketing ploys. In constructing a material-only dogma of human functioning, EBCM cannot account for our experience of conscious awareness, semantic meaning, pre-logical insight, preference, valuations, and many other body-mind-spirit realities that determine our health, wellness, and genuine happiness. Thus, when it comes to the EBCM healthcare model, our mental-spiritual properties are huge elephants in the EBCM circus tent.

EBCM research provides a statistical measurement for quantifying treatment outcomes in bell curve research findings. Quantification of treatment efficacy is then used to develop treatment protocols for particular symptoms or symptom clusters. Thus, in a somewhat simplified summary, patients enter the EBCM system and report symptoms or behavior in observable terms. Reported conditions are then rated by providers for frequency and severity and assigned a quantitative value. The conventional doctor then applies the material-only EBCM treatment to mask or suppress the symptom. An enormous fee is charged at the time of service irrespective of outcome.

As suggested earlier, the treatment plan ends up looking like a Whack-A-Mole game. Symptoms, like mole heads, are "whacked" when they pop-up. However, unlike the game, whacked symptoms whack back.

The "statistic masquerading as science" EBCM system has lead Benjamin Strong, MD to conclude that, "Patients have become victims of rote and standardized diagnostic protocols. The diagnosis of the individual has given way to diagnosis of the collective We now suffer terribly at the hands of the standardized protocol, or algorithm."[32]

Given that mole whacking can be so powerful that several moles pop up, it is easy to conclude that, from the profiteers' perspective, the more moles the merrier, mole whacking profits beget bigger and bigger mole-whacking profits. The mole whacking algorithm continues until the patient is bankrupt or dead.

Developing a science-based, body-mind-spirit health care system is our only path to ending the Whack-A-Mole EBCM game and plugging the profit-centric EBCM whirlpool that's sucking away our economic resources, destroying our health and environment. Such a system would eliminate virtually all the devastating health, economic, and environmental side effects of the EBCM medical system. By incorporating the data of our mind-spirit into our healthcare model, we can develop a reality-based body-mind-spirit science. Such a body-mind-spirit science of human health, wellness, and genuine happiness would not only revolutionize health care, it would shift the world from the unreasonable and irresponsible shifting sands of pragmatic EBCM to the rock solid scientific ground of our body-mind-spirit reality.

Any adequate theory of human health, wellness, and genuine happiness must, of course, incorporate the limited contributions of evidence-based research. However, we know that in addition to the limited value evidence-based research offers, all the components of a body-mind-spirit science are readily available and are being used in body-mind-spirit, science-based, medical systems. Naturopathic medicine is just such a science-based, body-mind-spirit system of primary care medicine.

Naturopathic medicine is the most powerful, effective, and safe primary care medicine available. Naturopathic medicine is cost effective and leaves a small environmental footprint. No one has gone bankrupt using naturopathic medicine. Naturopathic medicine is a science-based, body-mind-spirit medical system that works with, not against, our body-mind-spirit. The only barrier to universal access to naturopathic medicine is the EBCM profiteers.

Aware of the threat naturopathic medicine presents to EBCM profit-centric system, the profiteers have engaged in massive lobbying efforts and misinformation campaigns to prevent you from gaining access to naturopathic medicine. In the meantime, thousands of conventional doctors, without benefit of any training from regionally and nationally accredited naturopathic medical schools, knowing the damage EBCM causes their patients, attempt to provide "holistic" or "integrative" medical services. Conventionally trained doctors providing holistic treatments, is like an atheist becoming the Pope. In a nutshell, conventional doctors are not trained in natural medicine and have no business attempting to offer natural medicine treatments (See Appendix B for a comparison of conventional and naturopathic medical school training). It could be and, in my opinion, should be, considered malpractice. However, because they are "gold standard" EBCM trained, there are virtually no prohibitions on what primary care services conventional doctors can provide or claim they are providing.

The EBCM is about money. It's about eliminating or controlling fully credentialed, non-conventional professionals who offer more effective, safer, and less expensive alternatives than EBCM, so that the EBCM system can maintain its monopoly and profits. The effort has nothing to do with the quality of care. It is about protecting profits through conventional doctor oversight and control.

The next chapter will provide an overview of naturopathic medicine. The subsequent chapter will discuss emergent property theory, which provides the foundation for body-mind-spirit science.

naturopathic medicine
the whack-a-mole EBCM remedy

The damages and costs the EBCM system causes are like watching a tragic Mr. Magoo cartoon. EBCM blindly plows ahead seemingly unaware and denying or rationalizing all the destruction it leaves behind. The difference between the cartoon and conventional medicine is that while the cartoon Magoo is truly blind to the extent of the damage he causes, EBCM is not only aware of the damage it inflicts, it deliberately opposes and seeks to prevent consumers from having access to safer and more effective health care options. For all past, current, and future EBCM recalls by the evidence-based FDA think, "Oh Magoo, You've done it again!"

So, while EBCM commercials and advertisements shows happy images and suggest a happy life can be had by consuming whatever pill or procedure is recommended, nothing could be further from the truth.

What is being sought by such advertising is not happy and healthy; instead it is profits and maintaining a medical monopoly at the expense of genuine happiness and wellness.

What would be shocking then, is not yet another story by a conventional doctor like Dr. Oz, who seek the media spotlight by pointing their finger at their own profession, but rather a story told by licensed naturopathic physicians and naturopathic medical school administrators about the benefits naturopathic medicine offers and how naturopathic medicine can solve all three crises created by the EBCM system.

naturopathic medicine

Naturopathic medicine is a complete medical system that has a proven track record of providing superior primary health care at a fraction of the cost of EBCM. Additionally naturopathic medicine leaves a minimal environmental footprint. As stated above, the only serious challenge naturopathic medicine faces is the American Medical Association (AMA) and its powerful financial profiteers.

The miracle cure for health and wellness is not around the corner of the next consumer financed multi-billion dollar EBCM research project. It's right under our noses. The miracle cure for health and wellness and for resolving the acute chronic and catastrophic damage EBCM has created, and continues to inflict on our nation, is readily available. The solution is breaking EBCM's monopoly on the healthcare delivery system by licensing naturopathic physicians and other nonconventional healthcare professions in all fifty states.

Naturopathic medicine, unlike EBCM, is a complete system of medicine: It is not complementary, ancillary, or allied medicine as the AMA and its supporting financial profiteers would have the public believe. Naturopathic medicine rejects the science fiction of relying exclusively on evidence-based research for the development of medical treatments. Naturopathy operates from a broad scientific platform that recognizes the unique emergent properties of our body-mind-spirit. Naturopathy is at its core holistic in the sense that wholes are always greater than the sum of their parts. Recognizing our body-mind-spirit properties naturopathy has developed a system of treatments that integrates safe and effective traditional therapies with current advances in healthcare to provide a comprehensive range of preventative and primary care medicine.

The philosophy of naturopathic medicine is based on Dr. Henry Lindlahr's natural therapeutic writings,[33] which have evolved with our knowledge of our natural healing processes and now form the basis of the core curriculum at fully accredited naturopathic medical schools. Naturopathic medicine has a long history of preventative care, promoting wellness, and treating illness based on the laws of nature. Based on natural laws rather than a contrived, fundamentally flawed, easily manipulated "evidence-based" dogma, Naturopathic medicine is focused on the underlying cause of illness rather than symptom whacking, masking, and suppression. Focused on our body-mind-spirit health and wellness, naturopathic medicine is governed by the following Six Guiding Principles:

guiding principles

First Do No Harm: Naturopathic medicine uses therapies that are safe and effective.

The Healing Power of Nature: The human body possesses the inherent ability to restore health. The physician's role is to facilitate this process with the aid of natural, nontoxic therapies.

Discover and Treat the Cause, Not Just the Effect: Physicians seek and treat the underlying cause of a disease. Symptoms are viewed as expressions of the body's natural attempt to heal. The origin of disease is removed or treated so the patient can recover.

Treat the Whole Person: The multiple factors in health and disease are considered while treating the whole person. Physicians provide flexible treatment programs to meet individual health care needs.

The Physician is a Teacher: The physician's major role is to educate, empower, and motivate patients to take responsibility for their own health. Creating a healthy, cooperative relationship with the patient has a strong therapeutic value.

Prevention is the best "cure": Naturopathic physicians are preventative medicine specialists. Physicians assess patient risk factors and heredity susceptibility and intervene appropriately to reduce risk and prevent illness. Prevention of disease is best accomplished through education and a lifestyle that supports healing.[34]

The principles of naturopathic medicine are integrated throughout federally and regionally accredited naturopathic medical school training. The educational requirements for becoming a naturopathic physician are discussed below.

education

Naturopathic physicians attend federally and regionally accredited medical schools. The training provided is rigorous and comprehensive. Licensing requires passing both science and clinical board exams. The training received establishes naturopathic physicians as the only experts in the highly specialized field of providing safe, effective, and economical naturopathic primary care medicine.

Appendix A provides a chart that shows the difference between conventional and naturopathic medical school curriculums. If your conventional doctor claims to offer natural treatments, ask them about their credentials. Ask them what training they have received in "naturopathic therapeutics" and if they received their "holistic" training from a federally and regionally accredited institution. If they display an official looking "natural medicine" diploma on their wall check to confirm whether or not it's a mail order degree.

The main difference in fully accredited naturopathic medical school training and conventional medical school training is that conventional doctors receive no training in naturopathic therapeutics. They are taught virtually nothing about how nutrition, toxic chemicals, surgical procedures, or our mental-spiritual properties' effect on our health and wellness.

Conventional doctors do not even receive any training in the underlying philosophy of EBCM. The absence of EBCM philosophy course work is due to the fact that there isn't any underlying EBCM philosophy. EBCM is a dogma. EBCM rejects the fact that we have mental-spiritual properties. It is a dogma that disregards verifiable empirical evidence. EBCM rejects the empirical evidence that humans have unobservable mental-spiritual properties, insisting that all science must be observable. The non-observable data of our mental-spiritual properties, according to evidence-based dogma, is not only meaningless—it does not exist!

Conventional medical schools, bankrolled by EBCM profiteers, typically do not require a single class on diet or nutrition. School funding is based on training that provides the pharmaceutical illusion of health, while eroding your body-mind-spirit's ability to prevent and heal illness. The 7-12 minute conventional first office visit clearly demonstrates that pills and referrals for outrageously expensive procedures at controlling hospitals is what is taught and demanded by the EBCM system. The conventional first office visit has no time for your mind-spirit properties. If they offer any advice for mind-spirit issues it is not based on any evidence-based research and the advice they offer is most likely outside their training. EBCM training is restricted to using the material-only treatment required by the one-size-fits-all material-only algorithm to suppress or mask the reported symptom.

Conventional medical schools are not the "gold-standard" of medicine, health and wellness. The comprehensive training received by naturopathic physicians makes a huge difference in health and wellness. The difference is responsible for the incredible safety record naturopathic medicine has compiled over the last 100 years in providing the safest, most effective primary care medicine available, evidenced by the lowest malpractice rates of any physician specialty. Naturopathic medicine is the gold standard of medicine, health and wellness. EBCM is not even in the health and wellness game.

naturopathic treatments

Naturopathic physicians (NDs) provide primary care medicine to patients of all ages. NDs see patients with acute and chronic conditions. NDs employ all necessary diagnostic tools including physical examination, laboratory tests, and imaging. NDs may utilize physical and laboratory procedures to assess nutritional status, metabolic function, and/or toxic load, while considerable time may also be spent assessing mental, emotional, social and spiritual status to assure the treatment plan is comprehensive.

NDs use a variety of therapies to promote health and treat disease including: dietetics, therapeutic nutrition, botanical medicine, enzymes, physical medicine, naturopathic manipulative therapy, lifestyle counseling, exercise therapy, homeopathy, psychological counseling, and hydrotherapy. NDs perform minor office procedures appropriate to a primary care setting, and are trained to prescribe most standard drugs in the rare instance they are indicated. NDs collaborate with nurses and medical assistants and refer to specialists when appropriate.[35]

Fully accredited naturopathic medical school curricula, in addition to providing rigorous class work and clinical training, focus on therapies proven to work with the natural laws that heal our body-mind-spirit when ill and promote sustainable health. Conventional doctors claiming to practice holistic or natural medicine cannot begin to understand the complexities by taking weekend courses or reading an Internet article or getting a mail order diploma. They get away with claiming to be trained because their lobby has manipulated the state licensing boards to given them a virtually unlimited scope of practice. In any other field this would be considered fraud and deceit. In fact, they go after other licensed practitioners for any minor claim that impinges on their God-given monopoly. So without any accredited training in naturopathic therapeutics, conventional doctors are free to provide "natural" treatments based on the latest Internet article they've read. Moreover, with little training in monitoring emotional and cognitive functioning, conventional primary care doctors, often based on a 7-12 minute first office visit, prescribe close to 90% of all psychiatric medications.

specificity vs. comprehensiveness

The narrow and simplistic approach of EBCM is apparent across a wide range of activity. The conventional approach, isolating what appears to be an active material ingredient from its supporting components, and applying a toxic chemical to the isolated material target, is pervasive in pharmacology. Naturopathy, in contrast, demands, a comprehensive and systematic view of the person. The naturopathic approach, in recognizing that the whole is greater than the sum of its parts, in only the rarest of situations, would consider a limited conventional treatment beginning with the least toxic.

Focused on the whole person, naturopathic physicians differentiate how our whole body-mind-spirit experience affects our wellness. Based on the data generated from the 90-minute first office adult visit, physical, lab work, and other data as needed, naturopathic physicians diagnose and treat illness far more precisely than EBCM practitioners.

For example, a recently popularized, evidence-based FDA endorsed "food pyramid" stresses grains, vegetables, and fruits—

something naturopaths have been endorsing for over 100 years. However, the FDA's evidence-based food pyramid is a product of the reductionist paradigm that demonstrates a very surface and bell curve understanding of nutrition. The evidence-based FDA food pyramid lacks specificity to issues such as whole food complexity, food producing, processing impact, and an individual's unique physiology. A naturopathic physician, for example, is trained to further differentiate between whole grains and processed grains, between hybrid grains (semolina wheat) and naturally occurring "heirloom" grains (spelt), between reliance on a small number of grains, vegetables and fruits, and eating a diversity of fruits and vegetables. Lastly, the naturopathic community is appalled at the prospect of genetically modified organisms (GMO) and the negative impact such profit-based enterprises have on the sustainability of our health, environment, and economy. Notwithstanding all the evidence, the GMO do not increase food production, are not recognized by our DNA resulting in serious health issues, and are basically a get rich scheme. GMO profiteers are systematically killing off honeybees, monarch butterflies, and hoards of other insects and organisms critical to our very survival. For example, 30% of beehives collapse every year. Bees need biodiversity, Monsanto needs billions of dollars, so it destroys biodiversity by pushing one GMO plant for millions and millions of acres.

Moreover, naturopathic physicians not only work to develop diets and lifestyles based on each patient's unique needs, they also teach their patients how the digestive tract works to ensure what is eaten is absorbed. Additionally, naturopathic physicians often help patients avoid over-the-counter medications full of toxic ingredients that damage the body while masking and suppressing symptoms.

While a single toxic chemical can lead to health and environmental problems, the thousands of toxic chemicals we are exposed to on a daily basis in our food, air, and water are a constant threat to our health, economy, and environment. Again, using the honeybee example, in addition to the dramatically increased insect killing chemicals genetically engineered into GMO, honeybees have been found to suffer from well over 30 deadly human-made poisons. It's the combination of toxins that is killing our planet and us. These seemingly "obsessive" distinctions are not at all obsessive. They are all subordinated to the integrating principle of eating food and using products that have evolved in relationship with our body-mind-spirit and our environment over centuries in a mutually supportive and nurturing manner.

How do naturopathic physicians accomplish the critical task of creating comprehensive and individualized wellness and treatment plans for their patients? In addition to their five-year fully accredited medical training focused on naturopathic therapeutics, they take the time to thoroughly know each of their patients through the interactions that take place in the initial 70-90 minute first office visit. T is an example of a first office visit.

T, a 27-year-old female, is another example of how effective a 90-minute visit can be. T had a car accident eight months prior to visiting our office. She came in due to nightmares about the accident that were preventing her from sleeping. Her nightmares were vivid, intense, and focused on dying. She felt she was lucky to be alive, having barely escaped death. She had collided with a semi-truck and her car was totaled. She does not know how she came out alive and felt she should have died. It was a violent crash and she walked away with only minor physical injuries, but was emotionally traumatized. While she was exhausted from the lack of sleep, emotionally distraught, and on the verge of being unable to work, she did not want to be put on antidepressants or other psychological drugs.

I listened to her story. The way she spoke revealed that she was in shock about what had happened to her. She was reliving the accident over and over again. I gave her a homeopathic remedy and within a week she was sleeping again and the nightmares were gone.

If she had followed the conventional approach, her life would have been filled with anti-depressants, sleeping pills, other toxic psychotropics, and years of therapy. It is possible she would have been unable to work, ending up on disability. Under naturopathic treatment not only was she able to continue working, her healthcare costs were minimal and she is planning on going back to school to get her master's degree.

A, a 26-year-old male, is an example of how effective spending ninety minutes getting to know a patient can be. The 90-minute visit, in addition to the lab data, allows the physician to gather a great deal of body-mind-spirit information. The trained physician learns about the patient's life experiences and how their experiences affect their decision-making processes, lifestyle patterns, diet, coping strategies, and a wide range of other core issues that directly impact the patient's body-mind-spirit health. Most importantly, while the visit often demands enduring emotional discomfort by both the patient and physician, the patient often gains a great deal of insight into their body-mind-spirit disease and what they need to do to move toward the connected pole of the alienation-connected wellness continuum. The process, while often emotionally painful and demanding, has a powerful body-mind-spirit healing effect. The patient, often for the first time in a healthcare setting, feels connected by gaining self-understanding and being understood by another human being.

A was brought to me by his parents. He barely graduated from college due to extreme anxiety. After graduation he moved back home and for three years barely left his room. He was unable to drive, had difficulty even being in a car, and could not work or even think of having a job. He was up late at night and slept during the day. He told his long-term girlfriend to leave him because he was really "messed up" and she deserved better. He knew he was in a dire situation and agreed to let this parents bring him to our clinic. He told me that it took everything for him to come to our clinic, but he knew if he did not he would never get better and he desperately wanted to get better.

Our first visit was intense. I reassured him that I would help him as much as I could, but that he also had to work hard to change his diet, sleeping habits, decision-making process, and would need to take a few targeted supplements.

A was very compliant and worked to improve his diet, which was severely nutrient deficient. His parents also worked hard to support the changes and bought the food I recommended. They purchased the recommended supplements and the homeopathic remedy. We also worked on establishing a normal sleep pattern and shifted his decision-making process from defending against the discomfort of anxiety to identifying, understanding and embracing reasonable and responsible action.

Within a month, A started to come out of his room and engage in conversation. He started to leave the house to go to the store, which is something he had not done for three years. He started to visit his girlfriend's house more frequently. Within two months he started to drive himself to his girlfriend's house. His parents were amazed at the change and supported his progress.

Today, A has a job, drives himself to work, and has a baby with his girlfriend. He is able to participate in life and is no longer locked up in his room. He is a confident and attentive father.

As in the case of A, we need to approach our body-mind-spirit health from many data points. By examining a good comprehensive case, it is easy to see that poor quality sleep, poor nutrition, lack of exercise, and decision-making processes all need to be addressed to support proper body-mind-spirit health.

Homeopathy, which can play a pivotal role in resolving complex cases, requires taking an in-depth case study and carefully listening to the patient. Once the patient feels understood and connected, the healing begins. It takes time and patience getting to know and understand the patient. This cannot be done in an average 7-10 minute conventional doctor visit.

the first office body-mind-spirit visit

The first office visit with a naturopathic physician, in contrast to the 7-12 minute first conventional doctor visit, lasts 70-90 minutes, costs far less than a conventional visit, and rarely results with a referral to a profit-centric conventional hospital. During the first office visit, the naturopathic physician completes a physical exam, conducts a complete and comprehensive case history, and orders comprehensive blood work labs. Additionally, the patient is asked extensive questions about their diet, lifestyle, and emotional and cognitive functioning—with a focus on stressors. Together, the observable and subjective data gathered provide the naturopathic physician with the body-mind-spirit data essential to begin considering treatment options.

What many naturopathic patients report after their first appointment is a wide range of physical, mental, and spiritual benefits simply from being understood for the first time in the course of the intense 70-90-minute first office visit. They also leave with a number of safe nontoxic preliminary treatments and recommendations. Typically, a 30-minute return visit is scheduled to allow the naturopathic physician the opportunity to review any laboratory work ordered and spend the time necessary to develop a comprehensive and individualized treatment plan based on the body-mind-spirit data collected and analyzed.

It should be noted that the cost structure of conventional medicine simply cannot sustain anything thing beyond a 7-12-minute first office visit. It also demands the use of pharmacology, unnecessary testing, and unnecessary hospital visits, all needed to pay for the unnecessary medical equipment, summer homes, and fancy cars conventional doctors are entitled to. It should be noted that the vast majority of conventional doctors and conventional medicine clinics are either owned, or have exclusive contracts with, a hospital system. They refer to the hospital and the hospital refers to them.

Michelle A. Brannick, ND, DC:
my path to body-mind-spirit health wellness

It was my poor health that drove me to seek answers. I became the physician I needed—the physician we all need. I was 21 years old and was experiencing severe pain throughout my body, particularly in my lower legs. I needed crutches to walk. Prior to the onset of this pain I was athletic; I had earned a brown belt in Taekwondo and ran several times a week. I really pushed my body. In addition to Taekwondo and running, I waited tables several nights a week working my way through college. The debilitating pain I was experiencing affected every aspect of my life. I eventually had to quit my waitress job and all my athletic activities. I became inactive and depressed.

After seeing several doctors, all of whom just gave me pain medication or muscles relaxants, I was still in chronic severe pain and not getting any better. Not one of them (including those at a famous clinic in Minnesota) ever asked me what I ate. Because they could not help me, they started to tell me that it was all in my head. I remember thinking, how absurd! They thought at the age of 21 I wanted to become debilitated and quit all the things in life I loved! Yet I hear this "all in your head diagnoses" frequently from patients who have health difficulties that are not easily masked by drugs or surgeries.

As I drove home crying and feeling hopeless after one of my doctor appointments, I knew I had to take matters into my own hands. I was about to graduate from college. I had earned a degree in mathematics and statistics with a minor in physics. I knew I had to figure this out on my own or my life would be one of pain, misery, and despair.

I never heard a single word about nutrition from the conventional doctors I had seen but started to read about nutrition. I changed my diet relatively quickly. My eating habits throughout college were horrible, however, at that time I had no idea how negatively they were affecting my health. Now that I am a naturopathic physician, I understand what I did to my body! My diet was all fast food, all processed food (filled with over 5,000 chemical additives allowed by the FDA), soda, candy bars, and just about every other type of junk food. I rarely ate a vegetable or fruit in those four years, nor did I ever drink pure water! I felt like a honeybee choking on the products of our profiteer-created Pleasure Island toxins. Needless to say, as I improved my diet, my health improved and my pain decreased.

After college, I went to work as an insurance underwriter and then, after receiving a massage given me as a gift from my parents, I became interested in massage therapy. My transition from the conventional medical mindset to the natural mindset deepened while attending massage school. That was a major turning point in my life. I was exposed to many different forms of medicine in the naturopathic field and, of course, the healing power of touch. I continue to use massage and various forms of it today in my practice. Most forms of medicine look for and treat the cause of illness, except for conventional medicine. This idea fascinated me and I had to learn more.

It took me 10 years to get my health 80% better. Every now and then I would feel that leg pain again and I just wanted it gone permanently. I started taking some supplements. However, at that time, since conventional doctors are not required to take a single class on nutrition, and I was not aware of naturopathic medicine, I did not receive any advice about diet and nutrition. So my recovery was slow lacking professional guidance. How I wish I would have known about naturopathic medicine back then.

I eventually went to naturopathic medical school and became a naturopathic physician. Once I started this amazing education, I restored my health to 100 percent. I now can do for others in six months what took me over ten years to do for myself. I've become the doctor I needed then and now I can help others seeking to heal themselves.

Currently, I am in perfect health. I work 10-12 hours a day, six days a week, helping my patients live healthy and meaningful lives. I am very particular with what I put into my body. I do not recommend things to my patients I will not take myself. I live life to its fullest and have more energy and vitality than I did at age 21. I healed my body completely naturally. I have not taken an antibiotic, pain medication, over-the-counter, or prescription drug for over 25 years. As a naturopathic physician, I take the time to treat the underlying cause of dysfunction rather than mask or suppress it. In the vast majority of cases this is the only truly safe and effective way to heal the body-mind-spirit.

The mistake most patients make is to suppress symptoms with antihistamines, antidepressants, pain medications, or steroids, just to name a few. Suppression and hiding symptoms are not health. A lack of symptoms is not health. Health is living life with vitality and mental clarity, which requires the optimal and unencumbered functioning of every cell in the body. I want others to know there are many ways to heal the body-mind-spirit when given a supportive environment. To start the process we need to allow the body-mind-spirit to express its symptoms so we can figure out the underlying cause and begin the healing process.

Supporting the body-mind-spirit so that illness can be prevented and healing can occur requires a detailed understanding of each patient's unique physiology, lifestyle patterns (including diet and their eating mechanics), stressors, and a whole host of other factors that both individually and together impact wellness. Given the impossibility of providing a general protocol that would work for any two patients,

I have outlined some general treatment considerations that might be used for some common illnesses. Again, every treatment plan is based on the lab work data for each individual and all the other data points gathered from the extensive time spent with each patient and the individual specific information gathered from the clinical interview and other resources.

Thus, the treatment plans are provided for illustrative purposes only. In actual practice, each patient has unique physical, mental, and spiritual concerns, therefore, each patient, based on any number of factors or a single factor, might require dramatically different treatment approaches. Naturopathic medicine is not a protocol, or one size fits all, system of medicine. Patients are treated based on their uniqueness.

However, it is hoped that the following examples of treatment plans for some common illness will provide a general understanding of what a naturopathic treatment plan might look like. Additional information on the treatment plans for other illnesses can be found at brannickclinic.com.

common illnesses and non-toxic treatments

Fever

While naturopathy works with nature, conventional medicine, in contrast, typically distrusts nature, and often employs treatments that interfere or obstruct our natural healing processes. One of these natural processes is fever, an increase in temperature created by the body to eliminate pathogens such as harmful bacteria and viruses. We have been taught by conventional medicine that fever is harmful and needs intervention. Naturopathy acknowledges fever as part of the healing wisdom of the body-mind-spirit and welcomes the fever. It is one of the body's natural and best defense systems. Fevers give us an indication that the body is activated and working to heal itself.

Many conventional doctors are taught to artificially force the body to lower its temperature with medications, which can interfere with the body's ability to heal itself and can worsen the situation by allowing the toxic bacteria to propagate, not to mention creating a whole set of additional problems by the use of toxic drugs. When a fever is suppressed, the illness is prolonged. Because the body's natural process to destroy the bacteria has been eroded by the medication, there is an increased probability that the pathogen has not been killed off. The pathogen lies dormant or mutates and then resurfaces weeks to months later, whenever the body is weakened or compromised to the benefit of the pathogen. All this leaves the body in a more vulnerable state for more serious infections to occur. The misuse of antibiotics has led to the development of superbugs, which have created a serious health care crisis with the high probability of worsening to catastrophic levels.

Fevers are the result of an intentional mechanism by the hypothalamus (an area of the brain) to create an unfavorable environment for pathogens (germs) to inhabit. This increase is carefully regulated by feedback mechanisms to the brain, and the fever does not rise above 105°F unless there is brain damage, heat stroke, or poisoning. The degree of a fever does not indicate the severity of the illness. Once the pathogen is no longer a threat the fever retreats. Not only does the increase in temperature create an unfavorable environment for pathogens to grow, changes in blood composition occur. The iron and zinc levels are lowered and the copper levels are increased. Bacteria need iron and zinc to multiply. With a decrease in the availability of iron and zinc, the bacteria cannot grow. Fever also enhances the activity of the white blood cells particularly macrophages, so fever improves immunity. Fevers should be supported with proper hydration.

The occurrence of a "convulsion or seizure" associated with a high fever is extremely rare and is a grossly amplified fear. Dr. Mendelsohn, MD points out in his book, *Raising a Healthy Child in Spite of Your*

Doctor,[36] that after seeing tens of thousands of children, he has seen only one fever over 106°F. He explains it was not the high temperature that caused the convulsion, but rather an extreme, rapid increase probably due to a child whose health was compromised and unable to regulate the temperature. He also states he has not seen any permanent damage from a convulsion or seizure. However, he has seen damage in children who have been treated with anti-seizure medications to prevent seizures. Brain damage only occurs in a child that is susceptible and had a serious brain trauma where the hypothalamus that regulates fever is damaged and can no longer regulate body temperature. Higher temperatures above 106°F are seen in heatstroke and heat poisoning, which are medical emergencies.

Once a fever begins a child will get chills, which is the way the body generates heat (macrophages are activated). The fever is then sustained for a few hours to a few days. In babies the temperature of their fever will vacillate greatly. The duration and intensity of the fever is regulated by feedback from the body, which should be monitored but rarely interfered with. Once the pathogen is killed the temperature will go down automatically. As the body is getting rid of the excess heat, the child will sweat and look flushed. The way the body releases this heat is through vasodilation (vessels widen and there is increased blood flow to the surface of the skin). Heat is then radiated outward and the child starts to become active again. This process is the same in adults who generate a fever when they become ill.

There are so many ways to help a child through a fever, while supporting the body's natural defense mechanisms. If doctors spent the time educating parents about the damage they do to the body when they artificially suppress a fever I believe they would be more comfortable supporting the body to do what it does best. We all want what is best for our children, but sometimes it is hard to know when we are doing more harm than good.

Arthritis

Arthritis is an inflammatory condition. Naturopathic physicians and other holistic practitioners are educated to treat arthritis as a disease process involving more than just painful joints. Furthermore, naturopathy, being systemic (throughout the whole body), does not invoke a single, simple cause for each disease, nor a single, simple treatment. Ten people with the symptoms of arthritis may very well receive ten different programs of treatment. The treatment plan depends on the various causes of inflammation and the patient's specific strengths and weaknesses.

Inflammation is the body's way of reporting that there is a problem. It is a cry for help. For instance, when the skin is scratched the area around it swells up. This intense reaction is called inflammation. Swelling brings nutrients and white blood cells into the area to promote healing. This is a natural process and should not be suppressed. The body can heal itself if given a supportive environment. In chronic inflammation like arthritis, there is a continuous insult to the body that is not being eliminated. Therefore, the body is under a great deal of stress. There is a constant wearing down of the body's vital force and immune system. To decrease inflammation by taking steroids, anti-inflammatories, pain medications, antihistamines, or chemotherapy drugs does not solve the problem it just suppresses the symptoms and allows for the chronic insults to continue. The patient's health deteriorates as these medications harm the liver and cause damage to the immune system. The pain and swelling may retreat temporarily, however new symptoms often begin. If the cry for help has not been heard, the body will show its disparity in other symptoms and may even be named as a new disease when in reality it is the same process with a deepening of the original cause. Arthritic suppression occurs when the immune system is suppressed so that it is prevented from reacting to the irritants.

A relative of mine had arthritis and it was suppressed with steroids that damaged his organs, and he eventually died of organ failure. To properly treat arthritis, the physician must first stop all suppression. The body cannot heal and be suppressed at the same time. When suppression is stopped, the original symptoms usually return. Therefore, once the cause is identified and removed, inflammation retreats and healing occurs. This is where an experienced, skilled natural doctor shines. Removing suppression, minimizing symptoms, and supporting the healing process is both an art and a science. The art comes from experience. There is a balance between releasing suppression, allowing for symptoms to return, and promoting healing so the patient is in minimal discomfort. Unfortunately, if long-term suppression has occurred and there is damage to the immune system, long-term suppression may be the only option.

Conventional doctors may say they do not know the cause, so they need to suppress or mask symptoms. However, naturopathic physicians are trained to identify and treat the cause of inflammation. In addition, naturopathic physicians are trained to support the healing process and to identify, when and if, the treatment plan needs to be changed.

There are many ways to heal the body but it has to be given a supportive environment. To start the process we need to stop suppression and allow the body to express its symptoms so that we can figure out the underlying cause and begin the healing process.

Optimal health is an aspiration most people will never attain. Optimal health requires effort. A few people with excellent genetic make-up who consume a whole foods diet, exercise, and have a positive self-regard will experience optimal health.

Even normal health is rare due to all the environmental insults to the human body-mind-spirit. Most people, without realizing it, are used to living in a state of chronic illness. While test and lab results paint a disturbing picture, they report being in great health. Due to lifelong habits, exposure to our toxic environment, and impulsive negative behaviors, they have little or no experience of what great health feels like: In fact, they have rarely, if ever, experienced normal health.

Poor health starts with some type of irritation due to one or many insults to the body. This is the stage where the body is telling you that something is wrong and it is having a difficult time overcoming the disturbance. Symptoms may be a constant runny nose, post-nasal drip, fatigue, chronic cough, skin irritations, yeast infections, or genital discharge. Instead of treating the cause, we suppress these symptoms by taking antihistamines to dry the nose, cough suppressants to avoid coughing, Benadryl to control skin itching, and coffee to get through the day. In many ways we operate artificially by getting through the day on stimulants. We do not support the body to do its job. When the body tells us it is sick, we ignore it or suppress its cry for help. These little annoyances, or Twinkie Dilemmas, that we choose to ignore, mask, or suppress are a constant wear and tear on our vital force and slowly destroy our body's ability to heal itself.

A 38-year-old female, J, came to our clinic and could barely walk into the office without help from her parents. She was in extreme pain and her joints were so swollen she could not bend her knees, elbows, or fingers. Her periods disappeared three years prior to her visit. She reported chronic pain, fatigue, and poor quality of sleep (even though she was exhausted, she could not sleep). She took pain medications, however, they gave her very little relief. She also experimented with stem cell treatment and some Internet advice, but nothing helped her. She also had a rash on her forearm for several years that would not resolve. At the initial visit we improved her diet—her protein intake was too low and she was not eating the type of protein her body needed to heal itself. We provided her with anti-inflammatory supplements and support for energy and sleep. Due to the poor quality of her life at such a young age, she was also depressed.

Her laboratory results were as follows:

	Initial Visit	3-Months Later
RA Latex	788.3 (HIGH)	604.8 (HIGH)
Platelets	391 (HIGH)	281 (NORMAL)
Thyroid TPO	167 (HIGH)	89 (HIGH)
Thyroid AB	7.8 (HIGH)	4.0 (HIGH)
TSH	19.44 (HIGH)	9.24 (HIGH)
Vitamin D	36.8 (LOW)	46.3

Although her labs are not yet in normal range, the improvement is dramatic and within another three months we expect most results to be in normal range.

J is highly motivated to work on improving her health. She has a child who needs to be taken care of and a full-time job she needs to keep. She embraced her new diet and has been compliant with taking her supplements. After three months of her new lifestyle, diet, and supplements, her periods have returned, she is working out again, moving much better, able to bend her fingers and knees due to decreased swelling, walking without assistance, and sleeping better. Her energy has improved, her pain has decreased, her rash has resolved, and her mood has improved, all without the use of any prescription drugs.

We continue to work on her health. She stated that even if she stayed where she is currently at, she is so happy to get this far this fast! Natural medicine is extremely effective if used by experienced, professionally trained naturopathic physicians. She could not have achieved these types of results with the typical conventional approach. In fact, if she followed the conventional route, she was facing a life of severe joint deformities, pain, and organ problems from the side effects of immune-suppressing drugs and steroids. She knew this wasn't a healthy path and chose to try something different.

Acid Reflux

There are over 25 million Americans with heartburn/acid reflux/ GERD who spend over five billion dollars per year on antacids and proton pump inhibitors such as Nexium® or Prilosec®. Are those medications treating the cause of heartburn or suppressing the symptoms? The conventional approach is to prescribe proton pump inhibitors or antacids for heartburn or any symptoms related to digestion. Some patients may feel a little better, but are unaware of the damage that develops slowly while they are on these medications. Suppressing the acid may not be good for long-term health. Digestion is the function of breaking down food and absorbing and assimilating the nutrients. Proper digestion needs a high acidic stomach with a pH of 1–2 in order to properly break down food and to absorb minerals, proteins, and vitamins. Even a slight lowering of stomach acid or raising the pH above 3, prevents proper breakdown of food, which results in nutritional deficiencies. Antacids decrease stomach acid thereby decreasing the ability to digest. This results in undigested food traveling through the gastrointestinal tract and further irritating the lining and causing inflammation. Inflammation itself also prevents absorption of nutrients in the intestines, further exacerbating the problems.

Most digestion problems can be helped by proper dietary habits and natural medicine. Many philosophies of natural medicine believe that most illnesses or conditions start with weak digestion. Weak digestion equals poor absorption of nutrients, which results in weak organs, connective tissues, and immune systems. Weak digestion exposes the entire body to metabolic damage, which occurs when cells are deprived of basic nutrients. Organs and tissues, which are made up of cells, become weakened and ultimately lose their ability to function when our digestive processes become impaired. Digestion first becomes weak with chronic abuse. Chronic abuse can involve simple and easily correctable habits like eating too fast, consuming high sugar, high fat, and poor quality foods. With these insults, the whole gastrointestinal tract becomes sluggish. This results in symptoms such as heartburn, indigestion, gas, or bloating. Heartburn is rarely due to the common belief of overproduction of stomach acid. It is caused by a system that has been abused and has been weakened. The esophageal sphincter no longer closes resulting in reflux. Natural forms of medicine can strengthen the digestive tract when weakened. However, the insults need to be eliminated or decreased. We must change our diets and attitudes toward food. We must eat to nourish!

E is a 46-year-old male who was seen in our office for chronic GERD or heartburn. Onset of his symptoms started over three years ago and he had been on many prescription antacids, however, he constantly had discomfort in his GI system, burning in throat, burping, headaches, eczema, gas, bloating, constipation and fatigue. As his health declined he became nervous and anxious and his sleep became disturbed. He felt he was young and should feel better than he did, especially at his age.

He saw me after eight months of discontinuing all medications. His health had improved slightly, however, he was seeking more than just improved health; he wanted good health and good energy. We ran blood work and found out that he had many deficiencies. We changed his diet and supported his digestion with digestive enzymes and replaced the deficiencies.

He was willing to do whatever it took to regain his health. He was an extremely compliant patient and as a result of his willingness to do what was reasonable and responsible, he got the results he wanted relatively fast. Within three weeks of our treatment plan his reflux and heartburn was greatly reduced, he was sleeping through the night, he had decreased anxiety, his headaches resolved, his energy improved, and his eczema resolved. His bowel movements were much easier to pass, and he had decreased gas and no bloating.

When I asked how he was able to change his diet so fast, he said it was easy. He would do anything to feel good again. Nothing I recommended to him was a problem. He did what was reasonable and responsible for his health! E demonstrated the power of body-mind-spirit health, in that he sought out an approach that supported and healed his body instead of suppressing symptoms, which is the instant gratification pathway. Some of these changes may not have been comfortable, but he saw the bigger picture and sought to fix the problem.

By being reasonable and responsible, his desire to solve his health problems not only made him more productive in society, but also reduced his personal healthcare costs. Reducing healthcare costs allows for a significant reallocation of economic resources. This not only strengthened his personal finances, but also the national economy and reduced environmental pollution.

the science and art of eating

The process of eating is meant to stimulate the senses. It should be enjoyable as well as nourishing. We need to establish a reasonable and responsible relationship with food and how we consume food. Eating should provide nourishment, and not just be part of our daily routine. Counting calories creates a negative relationship with food. A calorie from an organic apple is different from a calorie from a Twinkie. Health is about the quality and nutrition of food—not about calories. Every cell in our body is counting on us. How we feel about food and eating plays a major role in how food affects our bodies.

Sitting down for a meal or a snack can be a time for regrouping our thoughts or enjoying someone's company. It can be a time to explore the senses of taste and smell. If the food we eat is of high quality, we can feel a sense of reasonableness and responsibility to ourselves—body, mind, and spirit.

Shopping for food should also be an experience that is rewarding. To buy fresh and high quality foods is to provide nourishment to every cell in our body. Shopping should not be done in too much haste, especially when working to improve dietary habits. Food should be bought and eaten as fresh as possible. The vegetables and fruit should look rich in color, not old and dried out. Purchase wild fish instead of farm-raised fish. Buy food that has the least amount of processing. Nuts should be raw and unsalted. Meats should be red without dyes, be hormone free and grass fed, and should be cooked medium to medium-rare. The key to healthy shopping is quality, which may cost a little more, but is well worth it in the long run. You are worth the expense of higher quality food and often the cost difference is more than paid for by lower healthcare costs. Avoid frozen or microwaveable food that provides very little nutrition and minimal stimulation of the senses.

Our health is vital to our well-being. Making time to cook can be quite rewarding and it reinforces the idea that you and your health are worth both time and effort. Meals should be eaten in a relaxed setting with the TV off, and in a sitting position (not standing up). The body breaks down and absorbs nutrients while in a parasympathetic or relaxed state. This should also be a time of family discussion without arguments. The food should be eaten in small bites, slowly and thoroughly chewed before swallowing. You may even decide to put the fork down after each bite to train yourself to slow down. The slower process will allow the digestive enzymes to work better, thereby decreasing heartburn, gas, and or bloating, while simultaneously increasing the absorption of nutrients.

Digestive dysfunction is a common side effect of how fast we eat and live. Our digestive system has not adapted to this new high-speed living style. When it comes to healthy eating, the number one rule is to slow down. When we develop reasonable and responsible diets and eating patterns, we dramatically increase the possibility of not only achieving optimal health, we become deeply connected to the reality of whom and what we are. With each step in the process from shopping to preparing meals, to relaxing and chewing each bite, we deepen our connectedness to ourselves, which allows us to deepen our connection to the entire universe.

antibiotics

Antibiotics cause damage to our immune system, kidneys, liver, stomach, teeth, tendons, intestines, vision, and nerves. Antibiotics should only be used in life-threatening illnesses, and are effective only for bacterial infections. Yet they are frequently prescribed for viral, fungal and allergic conditions in which they have no effect. The frequent use of antibiotics results in illnesses that are resistant to antibiotics. This means that if your body has difficulty overcoming an infection it will not respond to antibiotic treatments and will leave you vulnerable. Naturopathic physicians have been warning of this resistance for decades. Also, with chronic exposure to antibiotics, patients reach a threshold and start to experience side effects. I have seen many patients who have taken frequent and long-term antibiotics and think nothing of it, now they are chronically ill not even knowing it was their frequent use of antibiotics causing the current problems. The effects of antibiotics are accumulative.

Tens of thousands of people are damaged by antibiotics each year, yet most are undiagnosed or misdiagnosed. Our intestines contain 100 trillion different bacteria all living in symbiotic relationships with each other. The diversity of these organisms determines the strength of our immune system. The bacteria we are born with have developed over millions of years. When we subject newborns to antibiotics, we wipe out all but a few strains of bacteria and leave them compromised with weakened immune systems. The friendly bacteria will never fully recover even with the use of probiotics.

Most children receive antibiotics several times a year for minor problems that could easily be resolved by safer alternatives. The antibiotics used today are broad-spectrum and super-strength, whereas 40 years ago, small amounts of specific antibiotics were prescribed for short durations. There is a time and place for antibiotics, however, let it be known that our own children have never needed antibiotics and are in perfect health. However, if they contracted bacterial meningitis, I would give them antibiotics. Again, antibiotics should only be used for life-threatening bacterial infections.

Naturopathic physicians use vitamins, minerals, probiotics, hyperbaric oxygen, and herbs including berberines to overcome bacterial infections by supporting the immune system rather than weakening it. The net result is that the organism—the body-mind-spirit is stronger from the experience of having fought off the infection naturally and in a sense has "learned" from the experience.

D, a four-year-old girl, was brought in by her mother, who was exhausted by her daughter's poor health. At the age of two she had already been on many medications including steroids, antibiotics, inhalers, and antihistamines. Her mother felt that the medications were no longer working and, in fact, harming her health. D had ear tubes inserted and several hospitalizations, resulting in only temporary relief. D became difficult to handle, as she was very irritable, weak, and refused any more treatments. In fact, she started to vomit when given any medications. Her mother was seeking a different approach to restore her health. She was self-treating with Internet suggestions, but needed more help.

When I first met D, she was difficult in the office; she was irritable and demanded constant attention. She was very inflamed and had a wheeze, congestion, constipation, and fatigue with difficult sleep; yet she anxious and hyperactive. I recommended some herbs to detox her from past medications and to strengthen her immune system. I gave her mother some tools to work with at home and we changed her diet. The mother began to see that her congestion and wheeze would increase with exposure to certain foods, especially dairy products.

D's mother started to wean her off steroids and other medications as they were no longer needed since she was actually improving for the first time in her life. We started to rebuild her immune system with amino acids, herbs, and cod liver oil (anti-inflammatory). She was on a strict anti-inflammatory dairy-free, gluten-free diet. Compliance became stronger as results were noticed and the more compliant to her diet, the faster D recovered.

Within two months D was a different person. Her mother told me that she never knew her daughter and she was just getting to know her now that all the positive changes were taking place. Previously, it had all been about her being chronically sick on a daily basis and constantly putting out fires. Her child was now cooporative, sweet, calm and healthy! Even her teachers noticed she was no longer hyperactive in class and could sit still; she had productive energy and she was happy!

After just two months, she no longer had a wheeze or congestion and was having daily bowel movements. Not only did her mood and health improve, but it also helped the entire family. The family was under enormous stress due to the acute episodes. The stress also brought marriage problems and divorce was pending. After several months of progressive improvement, the family stress went away and divorce was no longer a thought.

Sometimes it is difficult to change course, but it is reasonable and responsible to seek the least invasive, safe approach in regaining health. The Hippocratic Oath, which says doctors "first do no harm," needs to be taken seriously. The first step is to seek the advice of a doctor specifically trained in naturopathic medicine at an accredited four-year naturopathic medical institution.

the naturopathic mystery

So, why might you be unaware of naturopathic medicine and denied access to naturopathic physician care? What are the obstacles to insuring that anyone who wants to seek healthcare from a fully credentialed naturopathic physician can receive the care they seek? There is only one obstacle and it is the powerful financial interests that profit from the EBCM system monopoly they have created and fiercely protect.

The financial interests that profit from the conventional medical system do not want you to be able to receive naturopathic primary care medicine. They do not want you to know that naturopathic medicine exists as a safe, effective, and less expensive alternative to conventional medicine. They do not want you to know that naturopathic physicians graduate from federally and regionally accredited medical schools. They do not want you to know that naturopathic physicians are licensed as primary care physicians in 18 states, many countries, and that they have an unmatched record of providing the safest, most effective, and economical primary health care available. They do not want you to know that naturopathic medicine leaves a minimal environmental footprint. They do not want you to have a choice in primary care. They do not want to lose their healthcare monopoly or lose one penny of their profits. They want you to believe that, conventional doctors with little or no training in naturopathy, are the "integrative" or "holistic" experts. Integrative means you have expertise in two or more distinct disciplines. Few conventional doctors have expertise in non-conventional medical systems.

Naturopathic medicine is a threat to the conventional medical system. Naturopathic medicine has a proven track record of achieving safe, effective, and financially viable primary healthcare.

The only serious challenge naturopathic medicine faces is the American Medical Association and their powerful economic allies.

summary
EBCM has become the leading cause of death in the United States, it is also bankrupting the nation, and causes a massive amount of

environmental damage. The overwhelming brunt of research clearly demonstrates both the inadequacy of evidence-based research for addressing the complex body-mind-spirit structure of humans. It has been proven that humans are more than simple material interactions. EBCM, based on its exclusive material-only approach, is incapable of addressing our body-mind-spirit properties.

EBCM proponents have not only failed to address the challenges that have resulted in the catastrophic damage caused by the practice of EBCM, they, through their professional organizations and lobbyists, continue to attack and bully competing medical professionals while conducting misinformation campaigns against other more effective and dramatically less costly systems of medicine.

We don't have to accept the deficiencies, dangers, and damage caused by EBCM and we don't have to accept the dangerous care offered by EBCM doctors who practice "holistic," "natural," or "integrative" medicine with little or no training, no accreditation, and no expertise. We have professionally trained and fully accredited primary care physicians who specialize in natural medicine. Naturopathic medicine has been in existence for well over 100 years. It is a system that has demonstrated unparalleled success in preventing and curing acute and chronic illness. It is a system of medicine that recognizes both the material and mental properties of human functioning, and has developed an integrative structure to address all areas of human health. It is a medical system with rigorous academic requirements offered through fully accredited universities. It is a system of medicine that, due to its safety record, is not encumbered by enormous medical malpractice insurance premiums. Naturopathic medicine is a system of medicine experiencing an unprecedented growth and demand. If quality of care outcomes and wellness are what matters, the reasonable and responsible choice is crystal clear: Naturopathic medicine should be the first option in primary care medicine.

Consumers need be able to choose what type of fully accredited healthcare they want. Based on the dramatic increase in the number of people seeking naturopathic options, the demand for choice is getting increasingly difficult for EBCM to suppress or mask. Once we are able to offer naturopathic medicine as a primary care option, we can begin to lead healthier and genuinely happier lives.

Additional information about naturopathic medicine can be found at the following Web sites: naturopathic.org; bastyr.edu; and brannickclinic.com.

The next chapter will identify what theoretical and methodological developments inform naturopathic medicine and provide both the science and methodology needed to overcome EBCM's exclusive use of evidence-based research. The chapter will explain how the whole is greater than its sum parts, Lonergan's Transcendental Research Method and the Rorschach Inkblot Method are capable of preserving the valid contributions of both logical positivism and representational theory, while providing the basis from which a fully scientific explanation of our body-mind-spirit can be developed.

Emergent property theory provides a unified explanation of the structure and operations of our body-mind-spirit.

Lonergan's transcendental method exemplifies a research methodology that integrates observable and unobservable data into a unified theory of our body-mind-spirit.

Exner's Comprehensive Rorschach System is capable of capturing and objectifying dimensions of our body-mind-spirit functioning. Together, these developments not only allow for an absolute understanding of genuine happiness, they also provide an absolute basis for understanding the meaning and purpose of human life.

emergent property theory

the whole is greater than the sum of its parts

G rounding genuine happiness in the innate structure and operations of our body-mind-spirit renders the EBCM approach as utterly inadequate. The essence of our body-mind-spirit is that it consists in inner qualitative, subjective mental-spiritual processes. You cannot understand our subjective mental-spiritual operations by observing the material elements of our mental-spiritual operations. Attempting to understand our body-mind-spirit by observing the material elements of our body-mind-spirit, as John Searle points out, is "like trying to duplicate the inner mechanisms of your watch by building an hourglass."[37]

EBCM's rigid dependence on evidence-based dogma prevents it from addressing our body-mind-spirit and the function our body-mind-spirit plays in our health, wellness, and genuine happiness. Emergent Property as the basis for human science, in contrast to EBCM dogma, recognizes the critical importance our body-mind-spirit properties play in our health, wellness, and genuine happiness.

emergent properties defined

An emergent property is a property that comes into existence or emerges from its underlying structures as a different entity. For example, water, which emerges from oxygen and hydrogen, is different from oxygen and hydrogen. It is the same for virtually anything in the universe; wholes are different, and more than, the sum of their parts. In respect to humans, emergent property theory accounts for how our mind-spirit properties emerge from our underlying biological properties. Understanding our mind-spirit properties as unique emergent properties, supported by our body properties, allows us to understand all there is to be understood about the human.

Emergent property theory stands in stark contrast to the reductionism of evidence-based dogma, which claims to eliminate our emergent mental-spiritual properties by reducing them to their material properties. Dunne captures the basic concept of emergent property in pointing out:

All... things—atoms, molecules, cells, animals, and humans— have one feature in common, their existence depends very concretely on the recurrence of a set of events... where there is regularity, we can expect to find higher recurring schemes dependent on the successful functioning of lower recurring schemes. We grasp each scheme by a direct insight into its functional relations and we grasp the whole conditioned series of schemes by a direct insight into how each higher scheme is functionally related to its lower ones.[38]

For example, our organs exist and are sustained by underlying tissue, which exist based on successful functioning underlying cells, molecules, and DNA. Emergent property theory, then, as Dunne states, defines all reality as a "conditioned series of schemes of recurrence that emerge and survive according to probability."[39] The emergent properties of biology, and biology itself then, as with any and all objects and events can be understood based on the innate or intrinsic intelligibility of their schemes of recurrence.

Intrinsic intelligibility refers to classical intelligibility (recurrent patterns or patterns that are repeated) and statistical intelligibility (patterns of probability and chance). Together, classical intelligibility and statistical intelligibility account for the recurring properties and natural laws that define any object or event in the universe. Thus, we describe objects and events in terms of their wholes as properties and emergent properties.

For example, apples have a number of recurrent patterns (classical intelligibility), which allow us to recognize apples as different from bananas. Apple skin, texture, and seeds are all recurrent patterns that define an apple. However, depending on any number of factors, no two apples are identical. The factors that make up the differences between apples are the statistical intelligibility of a particular apple that emerged from probability and chance. Emergent property theory provides an explanation of any and all properties of the universe. Emergent property theory accounts for how more complex properties emerge from and are qualitatively different than the parts they emerge from, yet are connected to the properties they emerge from. Moreover, emergent property theory explains how objects and events function, change, and develop.

In respect to humans, emergent property theory explains how our body-mind-spirit exists, functions, changes, and develops.

Gregory Bateson provides a detailed explanation of how emergent properties come into existence, are sustained, and evolve when he speaks of what he refers to as the stochastic process. The stochastic process, as Bateson explains, is a process in which "a sequence of events combines a random component with a selective process so that only certain outcomes of the random are allowed to endure."[40] Baking a batch of brownies is a simplified analogy of Bateson's stochastic process. When we bake a batch of brownies we can use a certain range of ingredients and apply a certain sequence of events to make the batter and bake the brownies. If during the process of making the brownie batter we close our eyes and randomly add ingredients, some randomly selected ingredients will work to create a new sustainable recipe while others would not. Organic dark chocolate chips, for example, increase the probability that the recipe will endure. However, if organic garlic were added the probability of the recipe enduring would, in all probability, decrease. Additionally, if chocolate chips were added, they would change the brownie outcome: The brownies that emerged would be different than brownies that did not incorporate the randomly selected chocolate chips. So it is with emergent properties. A stable recurrent pattern combines with a random property and the recurrent pattern continues, changes, and develops. Moreover, the added random component makes emergent properties qualitatively different from what previously existed.

Additionally, Bateson describes the operation of epigenesis as dependent on the stability of recurrent patterns in growth and development. In this respect, Bateson argues the "processes of embryology seen as related, at each stage, to the status quo ante."[41] Thus, as an embryo develops each stage of development depends on the recurrent pattern of the prior stage, just as the baked brownies are dependent on the existence of the brownie preparation and baking sequence. In comparing the development of a physical embryo with the qualitatively different mental properties, Bateson explains:

*The whole process of epigenesis can be viewed as an exact and
critical filter, demanding certain standards of conformity within
the growing individual.... We now note that in the... process
of thought, there is a similar filter that, like epigenesis within
the individual organism, demands conformity and enforces this
demand by a process more or less resembling logic. In the process of
thought, rigor is the analogue of internal coherence in evolution.*[42]

Mental activity, which is a product of all biological activity,
operates under the same underlying pattern as all biological activity.
The stability of logic is similar to the stability of recurrent structures
in biology and when a viable random structure or insight passes
through the filter of logic, development can occur. Thus, Bateson
supports the idea of emergent probability theory. He elaborates the
central issue as follows:

*In the stochastic processes... either of evolution or of thought, the
new can be plucked from nowhere but the random... In contrast
with* [reductionist conceived] *epigenesis and tautology, which
constitute the worlds of replication, there is the whole realm of
creativity, art, learning, and evolution, in which the ongoing
processes of change feed on the random. The essence of* [reductionist]
*epigenesis is predictable repetition; the essence of learning and
evolution (the development and ongoing existence of an emergent
property) is exploration and change.*[43]

Through stochastic and epigenesis processes recurrent patterns exist,
change, and develop. As development of both evolution and thought
occur, shifts of structural organization result in emergent realities that
can differ, and are more than the sum of the properties from which
they emerge. Thus, as Bateson concludes, "It is out of the random that

organisms collect new mutations, and it is there that stochastic learning gathers its solutions."[44]

Logical positivism's effort to reduce mental properties to material properties has no possibility of incorporating randomness or explaining emergent properties. Positivists can objectify patterns of emergent properties, but only as the mechanical combinations of pre-existing material elements. Evidence-based research completely reduces mental properties to material matter and thus has no way to allow for emergent realities or new coherent intelligibilities to be grasped and affirmed as inherently different from the mere combination of their material elements. The positivist explanations lose the creativity of the stochastic dynamic. Thus, through the pattern of emergent probability all biological entities are created, sustained and, can, given an appropriate random ingredient, change and develop. The human mind-spirit and, indeed, body, given that every biological molecule has a mental dimension, are examples of properties that have emerged from, and are different than, the biological realities from which they emerged.

All things and events that make up the universe of being, according to emergent property theory, exist as conditioned properties of recurrence, and are all interrelated. The properties are linked, both vertically and horizontally, to other conditioned properties of recurrence. Ecological systems are an example of how the biological world is connected.

In any ecological system the survival of higher-order animals is dependent on the survival of lower-order plants and animals. Moreover, all biological organisms in any ecological system are dependent on their continued connection to recurrent patterns, such as the earth's continued rotation. Such linkage not only supports the survivability of higher-level properties on the basis of the continued functioning of lower-level properties, it also allows for the restructuring of lower-level properties through the operations of higher-level properties.

In respect to human functioning, how we employ our mental-spiritual properties has a pervasive impact on all aspects of our body-mind-spirit. Evidence-based researchers sometimes refer to the impact our mental-spiritual activities have on our health as the placebo effect. The evidence supporting the fact that our mind-spirit properties affect our overall health is indisputable. Moreover, our body-mind-spirit cannot effectively function if it is obstructed by toxic food and pharmaceuticals.

The structure of our high-level body-mind-spirit properties is qualitatively different from that of the lower-level properties that support and condition the ongoing operations of our body-mind-spirit. Accordingly, conscious experience, the product of our body-mind-spirit properties, is an emergent and unique reality.

In recognizing that higher-level body-mind-spirit properties have a structure different from the lower-level properties, emergent property theory supports the claim that things are more than their parts. As Helminiak explains, "Things are not just their parts; things are new realities. Things are realities different from their parts and different even from the mechanical sum of their parts."[45] Thus, emergent property theory claims human consciousness, an emergent property of our body-mind-spirit, is not reducible to its parts and is different from the mechanical sum of its parts.

This chapter will now shift its focus to two specific emergent property theories, namely, Pert's information theory and Searle's biological naturalism. While in details and sometimes even in conception they differ from the understanding summarized above, in their general thrust, these theories support the claim that mental-spiritual functioning are emergent properties.

Pert's information theory

Pert argues that human functioning involves "a psychosomatic information network."[46] The mind, according to Pert, emerges from recurrent and ongoing patterns of information molecules or "neuropeptide" interchange. This information interchange according to Pert, "functions to link and coordinate the major systems and their organs and cells in an intelligently orchestrated symphony of life."[47] In Pert's theory, information interchange occurs as neuropeptides bind with neuron-receptor cells called legands. The interchange of information (mental activity) between the neuropepitides and legands results in "a multidirectional network of communication"[48] throughout the entire body. When the interchange of information crosses a threshold of activity, consciousness emerges with the capacity to discern the intrinsic intelligibility of, and assign meaning to, whatever we are attending to. In this respect, Pert argues, "when release and exchange function in their normative patterns, the amount of intelligence at work in the organism is optimized, orienting the organism toward reality."[49]

Mental activity then, is a process that can cut across all body-mind-spirit activity. Human mental activity, contained in Pert's "information molecules" operates on both tacit and explicit levels. Tacit mental activity operates without our deliberate conscious effort, while explicit mental activity, or conscious activity, building on and supported by tacit activity, operates through our deliberate mental or conscious activity. For example, employing tacit intelligence, we do not have to provide our body with deliberate instructions to instigate each breath we take. Likewise, a plant does not consciously instruct its roots to grow around a rock. However, when our biology reaches a certain level of activity, our explicit intelligence emerges and we shift from the zombie-like world of tacit mental activity to the conscious world of explicit or conscious mental activity. Thus, in operating from the explicit and willful world of consciousness we are responsible for all of our conscious actions.

Chopra supports Pert's claim arguing that information exchange within and between cells is directed by the intelligence contained in every DNA molecule. In this respect, Chopra states, "intelligence holds together the blueprint of each cell in its DNA."[50] Moreover, the intelligence innate to DNA directs each cell's internal activity and coordinates intercellular activity, which continuously restructures the human body. Thus, as Chopra concludes, "impulses of intelligence constantly create the body in new forms every second."[51]

This moment-to-moment restructuring of the body is similar to Bateson's epigenesis and stochastic patterns of evolution and thought and Lonergan's emergent property theory. In both theories, patterns of recurrence cause the emergence and continued existence of our body-mind-spirit while exposure to random patterns allows for body-mind-spirit restructuring. Importantly, obstruction of the normative pattern of DNA activity leads to body-mind-spirit health problems. In this respect, Chopra argues, "To lose intelligence is to lose control over the end product of intelligence, the human body."[52] Of particular note here is the toxic effect of pharmaceuticals, which often disrupt and can destroy the flow of intelligence throughout the body-mind-spirit.

Both Pert and Chopra argue that information, in the form of intelligence, tacitly operates at all physiological levels of the human and emerges as explicit knowledge at the level of conscious awareness. Searle's biological naturalism also claims that mental activity emerges from cumulative underlying biological activity.

Searle's biological naturalism

John Searle argues that consciousness is an emergent property of human biology that accounts for the unique nature of human consciousness. Thus, as Searle asserts, consciousness "is not a separate entity from my brain; rather it is just a feature of my brain at the present time."[53] Consciousness, then, according to Searle, is "a natural, biological phenomenon. It is as much a part of our biological life as digestion,

growth, or photosynthesis."[54] Consciousness, as Searle continues, "...
is both a qualitative, subjective, 'mental' phenomenon, and at the same
times a natural part of the 'physical' world."[55] Thus, Searle identifies
consciousness as an irreducible dimension of human functioning that
must be explained if human functioning, health, and genuine happiness
are to be understood.

Bernard Lonergan's account of human consciousness as an
emergent property provides just such an understanding.[56] In
Lonergan's analysis, human consciousness is an emergent property
that has a two-dimensional structure, which unfolds on four levels.
Lonergan's theory defines, once and for all, the structure of our body-
mind-spirit. It also provides the basis for developing a fully integrated
model of our body-mind-spirit. Additionally, Lonergan's analysis of
human consciousness provides the science for naturopathy's body-
mind-spirit healthcare.

Lonergan's structure of human consciousness

The next two sections will provide a brief overview of Lonergan's model
of human consciousness. Understanding consciousness is critical
to understanding body-mind-spirit health and genuine happiness.
Without our consciousness we cannot understand anything and have
no mind or spirit.

According to Lonergan, the two dimensions of consciousness
consist of a nonreflecting dimension and a reflecting dimension which
unfolds on four levels. In Lonergan's account of consciousness the
nonreflecting dimension of consciousness is identified as unfiltered
awareness of awareness. In contrast, the reflecting dimension of human
consciousness is identified as four-levels or mental acts, which allow us
to "turn around"[57] on our body-mind-spirit experience of ourselves and
our world, in effect allowing us to understand reality and assign value to
what we've come to understand.

nonreflecting consciousness

Nonreflecting consciousness is the most difficult property of consciousness to grasp. It is a unique property that while it is experienced, it along with all mental operations of consciousness, while providing the hard data of experience, cannot be observed and therefore it is not open to evidence-based research.

Moreover, nonreflecting awareness is such a unique reality that it is difficult to grasp through language. To wit, the structure of language can confuse our attempt to grasp our experience of nonreflecting awareness. In language virtually every sentence has a subject and object. However, in nonreflecting consciousness there is no object. In nonreflecting awareness there is only subject-subject awareness. Our awareness of awareness is not an object observed it only exists as experience while we are experiencing. Equipped with awareness, we are not sleepwalking our way through life or operating like a computer without knowing that we are operating and making meaning out of our operating. We are conscious and we know we are conscious.

We experience our consciousness and our experience of our consciousness provides us with data on our consciousness. The data we have of our conscious experience is data, and as data, our experience of our conscious experience is not only open to scientific investigation and explanation, it is essential if we are to develop a comprehensive and systematic, that is a adequate human science. Recognizing and seeking to understand the structure and operations of our non-observable consciousness is the only way we can achieve a closer approximation of what a human is.

The data of our conscious experience is not meaningless as evidence-based proponents would have us believe. It is, in fact, the most important data we have in understanding anything about anything. Without consciousness we do not assign meaning to anything. Without consciousness we cannot generate any idea or design, conduct, or interpret any research or common sense understanding.

In contrast to a computer (the evidence-based material only model of the human mind, see Appendix B), we are aware that we are aware or conscious. We are aware that we are breathing, thinking, sitting, standing, reading, etc. We are aware we are reading because, unlike a computer, we possess awareness of awareness, we possess nonreflecting awareness as a property of our consciousness.

Helminiak describes the unique nonreflecting dimension of human consciousness as "…not directed toward some object. It is not awareness of an object. Rather, it is awareness of the aware subject. It is awareness of subjectivity… this awareness allows the subject to experience him-or herself precisely as the aware subject."[58] Computers do not experience themselves as computers. Computers do not have consciousness.

The experience of nonreflecting consciousness is often mistakenly thought of as self-awareness, self-consciousness, or introspection. However, such conceptualizations miss the mark. Conceptualizations such as introspection imply a subject-object relationship. In nonreflecting awareness there is no object and there is no subject-object dynamic. There is no self or object being understood. The nonreflecting awareness is the experience of objectless awareness. In nonreflecting experience there is no understood dimension of the self. Nonreflecting awareness, as objectless awareness, is not, as Helminiak states, "something thought about. Rather, its content is something experienced. Its content is the subject's experience of awareness….This is the awareness that, in fact, constitutes the subject as a subject in the human sense of the term."[59]

Lonergan distinguishes nonreflecting consciousness by arguing that in self-awareness or introspective experience "what is found, is not the subject as subject, but only the subject as object; it is the subject as subject that does the finding."[60] Lonergan further explains that nonreflecting awareness is operative in human consciousness by the very fact that humans, in contrast to computers, consciously experience objects and events. Thus, as Lonergan points out:

> *Hearing is not merely a response to the stimulus of sound; it is a response that consists in becoming aware of sound. As color differs from sound, so seeing differs from hearing. Still, seeing and hearing have a common feature; for in both occurrences there is not merely content but also a conscious act.*[61]

Our nonreflecting awareness is, in a limited sense, like a mirror. A mirror, if it were conscious, would not only be aware of what it was reflecting, it would be aware that it was reflecting. Without consciousness mirrors reflect but do not know they are reflecting. We humans, through our consciousness, are not only aware of what we are reflecting or attending to, we are aware that we are reflecting and attending. You, the reader, are aware of not only what you are reading right now but also that you are reading. Our nonreflecting awareness, our awareness of awareness, in conjunction with our reflecting awareness are precisely the human properties which allow us to experience, understand, and assign meaning to our world.

Thus, while a computer can be programmed to respond to a sound, a computer has no awareness that it is responding to the sound. In human nonreflecting awareness, the act of hearing or seeing is a mental response. In this respect, Lonergan argues, "one cannot deny that, within the cognitional act as it occurs, there is a factor or element or component over and above its content, and that this factor is what differentiates cognitional acts from unconscious occurrences."[62] Lonergan goes on to point out that the content of any act of awareness, as differentiated from the awareness of the content, is that the content is "merely presented or represented, so the awareness immanent in the acts is the mere givingness of the acts."[63] Thus Lonergan affirms that "the nonreflecting dimension of conscious experience is "'he difference between conscious and unconscious acts.'"[64]

Again, in the case of the mirror, if the mirror possessed human consciousness, in addition to reflecting objects and events in its field of reflected data, it would be aware that it was reflecting those objects and events. Mirrors, because they are simply material, like computers, are not aware they are reflecting.

This review now turns to Lonergan's account of reflecting consciousness. Our reflecting consciousness, which operates in conjunction with our nonreflecting consciousness, accounts for the body-mind-spirit acts by which all human experience can be understood and valued.

reflecting consciousness

Lonergan's acts of reflecting consciousness are the key to understanding and differentiating Pleasure Island happiness from genuine happiness. In fact, it is precisely the acts of reflecting consciousness operating simultaneously with our nonreflecting awareness (and the whole of our body-mind-spirit), which allow us to differentiate the reality of objects and events from mere perception. Lonergan's acts of reflecting consciousness, in conjunction with the ongoing activity of nonreflecting consciousness, pinpoint the structure of human body-mind-spirit functioning that allows us to attain a reasonable understanding of reality and determine a responsible course of action. In other words, it is the source of our ability to know the genuine and authentic, the true and the good and to act in a manner that is consistent with what we know is true and good. It is the essence of our spiritual integrity that is to know the right path and take it.

Lonergan's acts of reflecting consciousness constitute the essence of our spirit, our capacity to know, and become connected to all that is true and good. It is a process that takes effort, and is often uncomfortable, but which results in permanent genuine happiness. In Lonergan's analysis of human consciousness, our mental-spiritual experience unfolds through "acts" on four levels of reflecting consciousness. Helminiak defines these acts as acts which:

> ...directs the subject toward some object. It is awareness that sets the subject over and against some object. It is awareness that attends to, reverts to, and reflects on, some object.[65]

The acts of reflecting consciousness allow us to "turn-around" on our subjective experience and make sense of it. The acts of reflecting consciousness allow us to make choices based on a reasonable understanding of the reality of our world. It is our choice to go to Pleasure Island or become fully human.

In Lonergan's theory the acts of reflecting consciousness or intentionality unfold in a pattern of conscious experience and questioning that define our innate mental-spiritual laws. It is precisely the acts of experiencing-questioning that define what philosophers, theologians, and psychologists have alluded to as the "spark," "force," "energy," or "spirit" that is guided by rationality. Our reflecting acts of questioning also account for our unique capacity to create lives and communities based on reasonable and responsible action, which results in the unintended consequence of genuine happiness irrespective of how uncomfortable the journey might be.

Lonergan's four-levels of mind-spirit experiencing-questioning (conscious awareness, understanding, reasoned judgment, and self-determined decision) identify the human mechanics of our human spirit. Lonergan's acts of mind-spirit experience and questioning are present whenever we are conscious. Present in any moment of consciousness, Lonergan's acts of mental-spiritual experience are transcendent. That is, the acts of our body-mind-spirit experiencing-questioning are present in all human experiences of consciousness—any time, anywhere, throughout human history, and across all human cultures.

At the first level of reflecting consciousness, Lonergan argues, "We sense, perceive, imagine, feel, speak, move."[66] The data we experience at the first level of conscious-intentionality is, according to Helminiak, experienced as "spontaneous question, marvel, wonder."[67] Awareness provides data and generates the experience of wonder, which spontaneously opens into a progression of questioning oriented toward correct understanding and appropriate valuation of our sensory and mental experience. It is the first principle in any scientific endeavor, any human attempt to make sense of anything. Questioning further promotes transcendent development (a central dimension of virtually any understanding of spiritual development) by shifting the focus of intentionality from the first level to the second. We move or self-transcend from merely experiencing to experiencing and understanding. We experience self-transcendence and become more.

Lonergan describes the second level of conscious-intentionality as "an intellectual level on which we inquire, come to understand, express what we have understood, and work out the presuppositions and implications of our expression."[68] As such, the second level of reflecting consciousness is characterized by inquiry and insight. Thus, awareness present at the understanding level of consciousness is, as Lonergan argues, "the awareness of intelligence, of what strives to understand, of what is satisfied by understanding."[69] Understanding, experienced as second-level acts of intentionality, as Lonergan further explains, "looks for intelligible patterns in presentations and representations; it grasps such patterns in its moments of insights; it exploits such grasps in it formulations and in further operations equally guided by insights."[70] At the second level of intentionality, questions of understanding arise and result in the emergence of insights and then conceptualizations, hypotheses, and theories. Finally, the insights generated further promote self-transcendent development by shifting the focus of intentionality from the second level to the third, rational judgment.

At the third level of reflecting consciousness, the insights, conceptualizations, hypotheses, and theories, which emerged at the second level are subjected to the demands of rational judgment. In this respect, Lonergan argues, "there is the rational level on which we reflect, marshal the evidence, pass judgment on the truth or falsity, certainty or probability, of a statement."[71] At the third-level of reflecting consciousness questioning such as "Is it? Is it not? Is more data needed?" emerges and confirmatory and contradictory data are applied to second level insights. Known contingencies in the subject's understanding of the attended-to object are pursued, bracketed, or identified as "get more information." The conditioned—that is, the as yet unresolved aspects of any explanation are reprocessed and refined through the "wheel" of conscious-intentionality until they are explained. Thus, Lonergan argues that third-level judgments of fact follow the law of sufficient reason. At the third level of reflecting consciousness, there is found, as Lonergan states:

> ...the effective operation of a single law of utmost generality, the law of sufficient reason, where the sufficient reason is the unconditioned. It emerges as a demand for the unconditioned and a refusal to assent unreservedly on any lesser ground. It advances to grasp the unconditioned. It terminates in the rational compulsion by which grasp of the unconditioned commands assent.[72]

The unconditioned simply means that all pertinent questions have been answered, and that the matter has been resolved. As Helminiak explains:

The conditions that prevented assent, the remaining pertinent questions, have been fulfilled, the questions have been answered. So a judgment of fact represents the achievement of a kind of the unconditioned, a grasp of the absolute sufficiency of an explanation, "This is it! All the pieces fit. No reservations, no contingencies apply."[73]

Thus, at the rational level of consciousness, Lonergan argues, "the link between the conditioned and the fulfilling conditions is a structure immanent and operative within the cognitional process."[74] The human capacity to understand and reasonably grasp reality enables humans to act either responsibly or irresponsibly. That is, we deliberately choose to act in a manner that is either congruent or incongruent with what we've determined to be a reasonable understanding of our experience. We choose to either eat the Twinkie or reject the Twinkie. Thus, Lonergan's fourth level of conscious-intentionality is characterized by questioning that which seeks to identify appropriate responses to rational judgments.

Lonergan explains that the fourth level of reflecting consciousness is known by acts through which we humans are "concerned with ourselves, our own operations, our goals, and so deliberate about courses of action, evaluate them, decide, and carry out our decisions."[75] Again, now that we know the Twinkie is unhealthy do we eat or reject the Twinkie? Fourth-level acts of reflecting awareness are characterized by questioning concerned with appropriate action. The question, "what can I do about it?" determines fourth-level acts of reflecting awareness. Having arrived at a reasonable judgment we deliberate on what course of action would be congruent with what we know to be reasonable. When we deliberately act in accordance with what we have determined to be reasonable, we act responsibly. Our consciousness is our self-transcending agency. Moreover, if we intentionally seek to embrace the impulse of our consciousness we increase our participation in the unity with all creation.

Lonergan's objectified operations of consciousness are absolutes of human knowledge acquisition. In this respect McCarthy states, "To call that structure into question intelligently and rationally is to presuppose its validity; to subject its principles to further questions and criticism is only to instantiate them in the course of critical performance."[76]

When our actions conflict with what we determined to be reasonable, we are irresponsible, and like Pinocchio on Pleasure Island we become self-alienated jackasses.

Again, using the mirror analogy, if the mirror possessed reflecting consciousness it could not only "turn around" on and understand the reality of whatever it was reflecting, it could also objectify the internal mechanics and process of how it was reflecting and objectifying.

We humans, through our body-mind-spirit properties, possess this very capacity. Our consciousness is the agency that enables us to objectify the totality of our experience. It is operative in any human effort to know. As Lonergan explains, "...the supervening act of understanding... is so central that to grasp it in its conditions, its working, and its results, is to confer a basic yet startling unity on the whole field of human inquiry and human opinion."[77] Moreover, our experience of our body-mind-spirit operations provides us with the data that are essential if we are to develop a comprehensive and systematic science of our body-mind-spirit. We don't have to change reality to fit the observable-only dogma of EBCM. We can develop a reality-based human science using the data of our body-mind-spirit by using the tools of our body-mind-spirit.

Lonergan's identification of the structure and operation of human consciousness, in contrast to evidence-based science elimination of our consciousness from "scientific" consideration, offers a comprehensive and systematic science for understanding how our body-mind-spirit determine our health and genuine happiness.

Based on Lonergan's work, our body-mind-spirit can be summarized as follows:

body

Our body is comprised of biological matter and systems. As biological matter our physical life form is bounded by time and space. Additionally, our physical dimension is primarily concerned with satisfying our physical survival needs. Examples of our physiological demands are experienced when we are hungry, thirsty or underwater and need to come up for air. The impulses of our physiology can have positive or negative consequences and our physiology can become ill.

psyche

Psyche is a mind property. Psyche involves most of what makes up our personality. As such, psyche is comprised of content such as our emotions, memory, imagery, and our values and preferences. Psyche draws from our sensory and mental data to let us know how we are doing moment to moment. Psyche's primary interest is to be comfortable within our body-mind-spirit and our environment. The patterns of experience, governed by our psyche, initiate powerful impulses to satisfy a number of desires we experience including pleasure, accomplishment, security, and attachment to others. The impulses of psyche can have positive or negative consequences and our psyche can become ill. In satisfying the desires of our psyche we can develop maladaptive beliefs, images, emotional responses and other content patterns that become habituated.

spirit

Spirit is identified as the cognitive dimension of human consciousness. Spirit enables us to replicate and judge the reality of anything we attend to, which allows us to participate in what is genuine and authentic. Our spirit does not contain any content.[78]

The purely formal structure of our spirit is contentless and transcendent. Thus, our spirit is not conditioned by time and space and, thus, our spirit cannot become ill or diseased.

Our three core dimensions, body-mind-spirit can be in sync or in tension. For example, we might find ourselves in a situation where we're hungry and we're in the presence of a Twinkie. In such a situation our body has let us know we're hungry and we need to eat to feel comfortable and indeed, survive. Our psyche, drawing from our sensory and mental data "tells" us we can satisfy our hunger by eating the Twinkie. So far, in this illustration, our body and psyche are in sync. However, our spirit in recognizing the negative body-mind-spirit impact of eating the Twinkie, "tells" us to manage our body-psyche discomfort, avoid the Twinkie, and find something healthy to eat. The message we receive from our spirit creates tension or discomfort between our spirit's demand for reasonable and responsible action and our body-psyche's demands to relieve our hunger pains and be comfortable. If we eat a delicious organic apple our body-mind-spirit are all in sync. We experience genuine happiness both in the moment and for the rest of our life.

How we resolve the dilemma is who we are, Pleasure Island jackass or attentive, intelligent, reasonable and responsible human. There is no such thing as a higher self or any other self for that matter. There's just us and we are the choices we make. Based on our moment-to-moment choices, we're either reasonable and responsible or unreasonable and irresponsible. When we choose to be reasonable and responsible, we deepen our connection with our body-mind-spirit and all that is true and good. In contrast, when we choose to act in an unreasonable or irresponsible manner, we become alienated from our body-mind-spirit and all that is true and good. The point here is that the demands of our spirit can be obstructed when we intentionally or unintentionally allow conflicting demands of body and/or psyche to interfere with the demands of our spirit.

Understanding our spirit is a critical component to understanding human health and genuine happiness. Given the central importance of our spirit in our health and genuine happiness, the next section will detail how Lonergan's model of consciousness accounts for our spirit.

defining human spirit

Before we can know if and how spirituality affects our lives, health, and happiness, we need to define our spirit. Our current popular and academic understanding of spirit is fuzzier than our understanding of happiness. If you were asked to define spirit what would you say? What evidence would you present to make your case? If you write your definition down, and then ask others for their definition of spirit, you'd probably end up with as many different definitions as the number of people you asked.

The confusion surrounding human spirit is found in both our common understanding and in academia. For example, shown below are a few popular and academic attempts to define our spirit.

> *"It doesn't matter what you call it—Spirit, Higher Power, Universal Source, Creative Intelligence, the Unified Field, Nature, or God— we're talking about the same thing. Plugging in to Spirit is the experience of feeling connected to some energy bigger than yourself."*
> —**Marci Shimoff** [79]

What does some energy mean? What is "some energy?" What if this undefined energy is evil? Shimoff's definition is fuzzier than a peach. Yet she claims our happiness depends on plugging into this radically vague understanding of "some energy."

> *"It is impossible to agree upon only one definition for spirituality... Spirituality is a word that has been used to describe the human need*

for meaning and value in life and the desire for relationship with a transcendent power…Spirituality generally refers to something that is transcendent, ultimate, and known in an extrasensory manner… and…Spirituality is a 'code word for the depth dimension of human existence.'"

—Fukuyama & Sevig[80]

Is it the depth of good, evil, indifference, or some combination of the three?

"I have used the term spirit to mean 'the vibration of nothing.' I know of no way to accurately imagine such vibrations. The closest I can come is through the notion of alpha (the potential to become anything). The vacuum is alive with these vibrations. They contain the potential for anything. The process for realizing anything, becoming aware of anything, results from reflection of these vibrations in the forms of waves. To accomplish this reflection some form of resistance that bounces these waves back in the direction from which they came must arise. How resistance arises is unknown."

—Fred Alan Wolf[81]

Holy moly! Not sure if I want to hang my hat on unimaginable wave vibrations.

"Spirituality is the 'courage to look within and to trust' what is seen and trusted appears to be a deep sense of belonging, of wholeness, of connectedness, and of openness to infinite."

—Shafranske and Gorsuch[82]

What exactly is within that we are supposed to be looking at? Is it the cravings of a pyromaniac or drug addict?

Spirituality, which comes from the Latin, spiritus, meaning "breath of life," is a way of being and experiencing that comes about through awareness of a transcendent dimension and that is characterized by certain identifiable values in regards to self, others, nature, and whatever one considers to be the ultimate."
—**Elkins, Hedstrom**, Hughes, Leaf, and Saunders[83]

What values? Hitler's ultimate world order? Any value can be used for good or evil. If I value being a firebug as the ultimate, is that spiritual?

"Spirituality 'is' a personal affirmation of a transcendent connectedness in the universe."
—**Eugene W. Kelly**[84]

What is the universe?

Not only do all the above definitions of our spirit lack any effort to offer a comprehensive and systematic explanation of "spirit," all the above definitions are purely descriptive. In fact, when I became interested in spirituality I was somewhat shocked at the lack of any systematic explanation of what exactly our spirit is and what properties humans might possess that could account for our spiritual experience.

If spiritual experience is a distinct human experience and if we possess properties that enable us to have genuine spiritual experiences, it is imperative that we secure a precise definition of what our spirit is. Moreover, if our spiritual experience is connected to something bigger than ourselves, we better know what it is connected to, how we connect to it, and what purpose the connection serves. While it's warm and fuzzy to assume that it is some warm and fuzzy wish granter and protector, it might be our worst nightmare. Jim Jones comes to mind.

Thus, while each of the above attempts to define spirit include some reference to commonly held beliefs about transcendence, connectedness to a greater entity, and an openness to the universe, none offer a comprehensive and systematic explanation of what our spirit is or what the external source we are to connecting is, or how we connect or plug into it.

In an attempt to build on the basic assumption of spiritual thinking, the Center for Human Development (CHD) claims to have identified nine criteria of spiritual development.[85] These criteria shown below are all accounted for in Lonergan's systematic analysis of human consciousness. Moreover, Lonergan's analysis is based, not on description, but rather on the structure of the human mind verifiable in our own experience of our consciousness and empirical data. Moreover, Lonergan's identification of the structure of our mind's spiritual dimension is open to comprehensive and systematic research. The Center for Human Development's nine criteria with a brief summary of how each of the nine criteria are accounted for in Lonergan's analysis of human consciousness are shown below.

1. **Developing Self-Concept**: Lonergan's self-transcendent dynamic of consciousness accounts for our developing self-concept. We consciously experience—we objectify what we consciously experience and thus change and develop with an ever-deeper understanding of our self-concept. The two-fold, four-level structure human consciousness enables us to experience, understand, judge, and decide in a relentless and ongoing process of self-transcendence, of becoming more and gaining a deeper understanding of our ourselves and our world.

2. **A Responsible Self-Awareness**: Lonergan's self-transcendent dynamic of consciousness not only accounts for our self-awareness, it is our self-awareness agency. Moreover, the structure of human consciousness defines responsible self-awareness.

3. **A Sense of Autonomy or Inner-Directedness, meaning a basic trust in the validity of one's own experience and values**: Lonergan's two-fold, four-level structure of human consciousness is oriented toward the true and the good, the reasonable and responsible. Moreover, the norms of our consciousness are the source of our autonomy, inner-directedness, self-trust, and the validity of our experience.

4. **Appreciation of Genuine Authority**: The self-transcending dynamic of consciousness defines what is genuine and authentic. Thus, genuine authority only exists as an embodiment of the reasonable and responsible and the source of determining the reasonable and responsible is our consciousness.

5. **A Principled Morality**: As presented above, human consciousness unfolds through a dynamic pattern guided by demands for openness, understanding, reasonableness, and responsibility. Such inbuilt activities define principled morality.

6. **A Person Orientation**: In which one places highest priority on relating to another person as a "Thou" rather than as an "It": Again, the self-transcending dynamic of consciousness oriented toward the true and the good is selfless in its self-transcending dynamic. It is fully present to the others and indeed, the totality of creation, as "Thou."

7. **A Holistic View of Development**: The self-transcending dynamic of consciousness guides all human functioning toward reasonable and responsible activity. Our consciousness permeates and influences all activities of our body-mind-spirit.

8. **Present Centeredness**: Allows one to live and encounter the richness and depth of reality as revealed in sacrament of the present moment. The self-transcending dynamic of consciousness is only concerned with the totality of what is genuine and authentic and only exists in the present moment. Our consciousness is our centering agent. It is precisely our consciousness, which opens us to the richness and depth of reality, moment-to-moment.

9. **Openness to the Mystical**: Lonergan: The nonreflecting dimension of consciousness contains data yet to be objectified. It is mystical in that the totality of its content has yet to be objectified and explained. Mystery is nothing other than surplus explanation. Moreover, it is precisely the "yet to be objectified" data contained in our nonreflecting awareness that accounts for our experience of being a part of something bigger. The bigger is all that has yet to be understood and objectified.

Lonergan's analysis of human consciousness grounds all nine of The Center for Human Development's criteria of spiritual development in human consciousness. Additionally, our spirit as a dimension of our consciousness, accounts for our capacity to potentially replicate the totality of the universe. Human consciousness, through its cognitive dimension (mental processes such as problem solving), is virtually limitless in what it can replicate and understand.

cognitive principles and human spirit

Completely unfiltered by the needs of our body and/or psyche, the cognitive properties of our reflecting consciousness are unbiased and unconditioned. That is, our cognitive properties are free to become anything, and thus understand the truth, goodness, and reality of the universe. That is, while our cognitive properties are absolute in structure and operation, the absolute structure of our cognitive operations account for our capacity to develop a reasonable and responsible response specifically tailored to any context or situation.

Blasi, in describing cognitive principles, explains the open-endedness of the cognitive dimension of our consciousness as follows:

> *Cognitive principles constitute the broadest and most encompassing structure that one can imagine.... But precisely because cognition is so general, so open to everything, it cannot contain the principles of its specific realizations.... What is principle of generality cannot be at the same time be a principle of determination.*[86]

Specific realizations are content, the stuff of psyche-dimension of our mental properties. For example, the formula of an isosceles triangle is analogous to the cognitive dimension of our minds, while a specific triangle is the stuff of our psyche. Thus, while the formula of an isosceles triangle applies to all isosceles triangles, the specifics or content of any given isosceles triangle only applies to a given isosceles triangle. In effect, the cognitive operations of human consciousness are unconditioned and unconstrained by pre-determined (specific) ideas, concepts, categories, or any other content. As Blasi concludes, "Cognition does not offer the principle of determination, of preference, of value."[87] Those are the products of our psyche; the content-generating dimension of our mental experience.

The cognitive dimension of our mental experience is not limited or biased by any filter or condition, it is unconditioned and unconstrained. It is precisely the freedom of our unconditioned and unconstrained cognitive mental properties that accounts for what has been described as the "free movement of our spirit." The unconditioned and unconstrained structure of the cognitive dimension of the human mind enables us to participate, moment-to-moment, in an unending process of genuine and authentic self-transcendence and relentless processes for participating more fully in the totality of the universe. It is through the unconditioned operations of our conscious experience that we experience insights and can gain a reasoned grasp of reality. Given the unconditioned and unconstrained reality of our spirit, religion and evidence-based dogma are human-created obstructions to the fundamental structure of our spirit.

The emergence of insights or awareness about some object or event, whether concrete or abstract, occurs through our consciousness. The vastness of our nonreflecting awareness is always well beyond what we can objectify, and expands further with every act of our conscious experience. Thus, as indicated above, Lonergan's model of consciousness defines the key spiritual characteristics of genuineness, authenticity, and morality.

genuineness, authenticity, and morality

Lonergan's model of consciousness defines human genuineness, authenticity, and morality. Genuineness and authenticity are actualized when we faithfully adhere to our inbuilt capacity to be aware, understand, achieve, sufficiently reason, and act responsibly.

While the Ten Commandments, the principles Steven Covey details in his *The 7 Habits of Highly Effective People*, and the Socratic method (Socrates method of questioning used to determining truth) are examples of how the structure of consciousness has been formalized into genuine and authentic guidelines for reasonable and responsible activity, our consciousness is the final arbitrator of the reasonable and responsible in any and all situations. For example, given the context of a particular situation, what appears to be reasonable and responsible or genuine and authentic from a generalized perspective, might be unreasonable and irresponsible. Thus, while the commandment, "Thou shalt not kill" is unambiguous, few would argue that it is not reasonable and responsible to kill if it means protecting innocent children from being murdered. The same can be said for virtually any "value" that is universally understood as good. Telling the truth when the intent is malicious is neither reasonable nor responsible, it is disingenuous, inauthentic, and immoral. Thus, while formalized patterns of reasonable and responsible action often facilitate the creation of deeply connected and sustaining relationships, genuineness and authenticity is a moment-to-moment process arbitrated by our consciousness, not a set of rules.

In my practice I offer another set of guidelines that have emerged from our consciousness. This structure is referred to as the five T's of successful relationships:

The T's are Time, Talking, Trust, Truthfulness, and Tenderness. As discussed earlier, values can be used for good or evil. A value, depending how it is employed, can be a vice or virtue. The status of a value turns on whether or not it is employed in service of reasonable and responsible actions as defined by Lonergan's four levels of consciousness. Thus, the success of the T's is determined based on their reasonable and responsible use given the moment-to-moment context of a given situation.

a paradigm shift

The identification of the content-less property of the human mind, oriented toward replicating the reality of whatever enters our awareness, resolves a number of centuries-old challenges to our ability to understand human functioning, change, development, and genuine happiness uncovered by representational theory. These challenges left unresolved have led to our capitulation of seeking a scientific understanding of our mental and spiritual experience and our exclusive reliance on the pragmatic use of evidence-based dogma.

Human spirit, as a property of human consciousness can be understood and explained. There is now both a scientific explanation for our spiritual experience and its properties. As a property of human consciousness, the spirit is fully human and it exists in all humans. As a human property, it is open to scientific explanation. Moreover, as will be shown below in the section on the transcendental method, there is a scientific method for validating the above claims about our spirit and providing the basis for developing a comprehensive and systematic human science. Thus, in contrast to Kant's a priori categories and Descartes' idea of innate human knowledge, McCarthy argues, Lonergan "...strategically subordinates metaphysics, semantics, logic, and epistemology to an antecedent cognitional theory"[88] In doing so, the foundations of knowing is not found in positivist "facts" or constructed concepts, but in the structure and operations of human consciousness.

Our spirit is housed in our consciousness. It cannot exist in any other medium. Without consciousness we are unable to know anything, assign meaning or purpose to anything, or experience genuine happiness. Without consciousness we become the zombie computers of evidence-based dogma. However, we have consciousness and our consciousness demands we become ever more deeply connected with the unity of all that is true and good. Positing our spirit in our created consciousness is not a denial of theism. In fact, it is a science-based defense of theism. To wit, a comprehensive, that is a scientific, explanation of anything must offer a reasonable explanation of the original source of everything. What creates, conserves, and concurs in everything in the universe created, conserves, and concurs in our consciousness. Human consciousness is unique in that its fundamental function is to relentlessly participate in the universe of being through its innate dynamic of self-transcendence. That is, human consciousness seeks an ever-deeper participation in God. Moreover, like God it can be experienced but not seen.

Lonergan's analysis of human consciousness gives explanatory power to the understanding philosophers and religious thinkers have held throughout the centuries, that human spirit is a vital source or inner spark directed by reason. Reason is the driving property of our consciousness. Lonergan's analysis of human consciousness provides the basis for developing a comprehensive and systematic science-based model of our body-mind-spirit. Lonergan's model of consciousness, along with the body of knowledge developed by emergent property theorists, provides the basis for resolving the challenges and gaps in the EBCM system.

Having identified the structure of our mental properties and how they emerge from our body, Lonergan used the structure of consciousness to identify a scientific methodology that integrates our body-mind-spirit into a unified science.

Lonergan's scientific methodology is referred to as the transcendental method.[89] In his analysis of consciousness, Lonergan identified the basic mental pattern of human consciousness. Thus, this basic pattern is transcendent. It applies anytime we are conscious. It is not constrained by culture or by an historical period. Moreover, the very structure of our consciousness provides the structure for a comprehensive and systematic human science.

transcendental method

Lonergan's transcendental method is based on the very structure of consciousness. Transcendental method is a given, it is the normal activity of the human mind which allows us to grasp the reality of any human instance of understanding. That is, in every instance of our consciousness we employ the process of the transcendental method. You can glance at anything in your immediate environment, conduct a sophisticated research project, or close your eyes and imagine being beamed aboard the Starship *Enterprise*. In all instances the very same mental norms are at work. Thus, as Lonergan explains:

> However true it is that one attends, understands, judges, decides
> differently in the natural sciences, in the human sciences, and in

*theology, still the differences in no way imply or suggest a transition
from attention to inattention, from intelligence to stupidity, from
reasonableness to silliness, from responsibility to irresponsibility.*[90]

Lonergan explains that the transcendental method, as the
very operations of the human mind, qualifies as a method in that
transcendental method, like any valid method, as "a normative pattern
of recurrent and related operations yielding cumulative and progressive
results."[91] Moreover, Lonergan argues that all valid methodologies
must be anchored in the transcendental method because any method
must involve more than a set of rules if it is to yield cumulative and
progressive results.

Cumulative results require a sustained succession of discoveries.
Progressive results, as Lonergan points out, are only achieved if there
is "a synthesis of each new insight with all previous, valid insights."[92]
This is a core difference between science and ideology and dogma:
Science must incorporate all valid data in its findings. The evidence-
based method is not a valid human science in that it disregards the valid
data of our mind-spirit. Evidence-based research cannot synthesize new
insights with all previous insights because it disregards all valid insights
in respect to the reality of our mind-spirit.

However, as Lonergan continues, neither discovery nor synthesis,
"...is at the beck and call of any set of rules."[93] While cumulative and
progressive, results can be increased by methodological rules, such results
as Lonergan points out, "cannot be assured by a set of prescriptions."[94] For
example, evidence-based research methodology is a set of prescriptions.
Therefore, Lonergan concludes, any and all methodologies must involve
"a prior, normative pattern of operations from which rules may be
derived."[95] To wit, human consciousness. The operations within such a
prior normative pattern of activity must include both logical and non-
logical operations. Evidence-based research and computer hardware and

software are purely logical. Human consciousness, on the other hand, is both logical (reasoned) and non-logical (pre-reasoned insight).

Thus, the normative pattern of non-logical operations falls outside of evidence-based methodology. The logical and non-logical operations are comprised of Lonergan's two-fold, four-level structure on human consciousness presented above. Within the structure of consciousness, and only within the structure of consciousness, are both the logical and non-logical operations of "seeing, hearing, touching, tasting, inquiring, imagining, understanding, conceiving, formulating, reflecting, marshaling and weighing the evidence, judging, deliberating, evaluating, deciding, speaking, writing" present.[96] Any scientific methodology addressing human nature must include the logical and non-logical operations of our human body-mind-spirit.

While validation of Lonergan's model of consciousness is possible through our experience of our consciousness, psychological instruments also offer evidence of the structure and operations of human consciousness. The Rorschach inkblot method is just such an instrument. In this respect, Exner argues that the RIM reflects the inner psychological processes that account for how we understand the world around us.[97]

summary

This chapter detailed how emergent property theory provides a comprehensive basis that can resolve the core challenges that EBCM faces in understanding what treatments work with our body-mind-spirit to reduce illness and support wellness.

Human wellness and genuine happiness involve the totality of our body-mind-spirit. Lonergan's model of consciousness, supported by the work of other emergent property theorists, provides a theoretical framework within which a comprehensive and systematic science of our body-mind-spirit can be developed.

Lonergan's model of consciousness explains what Rogers believed was a "tiny peak of awareness, of symbolizing capacity based on a vast pyramid of non-conscious organismic functioning."[98] This tiny peak of awareness, the human property that Lonergan systematically explains as the structure and operations of consciousness, has a pervasive effect on human health, change, development, and genuine happiness.

As the apex of human evolutionary development, human consciousness represents the highest integrating property of the human. Helminiak pinpoints the central impact that consciousness has on human functioning in arguing that "in humans consciousness opens onto a realm beyond biological life…consciousness expresses itself in the demand for the coherence of explanation, the consistency of fact and the endurance and validity of goodness."[99] In short, genuine happiness. To wit, Rogers insisted that human wellness is experienced when one is attentive to, deliberately embraces, and acts in accordance with his or her actualizing processes. On the other hand, maladaptive mental functioning results when one's actualizing processes are suppressed, repressed, denied or otherwise disrupted. This very dynamic is what determines our experience of self-alienation or connectedness.

Theories and research grounded on evidence-based dogma and representational assumptions exclusively focus on observable material phenomena by reducing wholes to their material elements. The material elements are then whacked with material chemicals or removed with little consideration of the operation of the whole. In a sense it is pornographic. Is exclusively concerned with the physical. Pornography is completely disinterested in the human mind-spirit. In the pornographic world there are no profits to be made from a victim's mind or spirit. In fact, consideration of a victim's mind or spirit is a threat to profits. The victims are mindless and spiritless commodities. Likewise, conventional medicine is exclusively focused on how profits can be generated by material- or physical-only research and treatments.

Our mind-spirit is explicitly viewed as meaningless. Moreover, as evidenced by the elimination from, and insurance or government payment for, treatments related to "subjective," that is, mind-spirit treatments, are not profitable.

Emergent probability theory, on the other hand, is focused on objectifying the reality of both the observable properties and the non-observable properties of the whole. Emergent property research exploits the full range of data available for scientific investigation. That is, emergent property research integrates both observable evidence-based research with non-observable mind-spirit data.

Lonergan's theory of human consciousness and his articulation of the transcendental method, provide both the theoretical and the methodological basis for a unified explanation of our body-mind-spirit. This explanation, in turn, provides the human sciences the foundation for a comprehensive and systematic understanding of human functioning, so that healthy change and genuine happiness can be developed.

Human mental functioning must be explained on the basis of our body-mind-spirit, rather than on the limited and distorting data of evidence-based research. Therefore, to grasp the structure and operations of human mental functioning, one must experience the structure and operations of human mental functioning. The structure and operations of human mental functioning are there to be known: One need only attend to them. Go ahead give it a try. You can do it! To increase the likelihood of success, as Lonergan explains:

> One raises the level of one's activity. If one sleeps and dreams, one is present to oneself as the frightened dreamer. If one wakes, one becomes present to oneself, not as moved but as moving, not as felt but as feeling, not as seen but as seeing. If one is puzzled and wonders and inquires, the empirical subject becomes an intellectual subject as well. If one reflects and considers the

evidence, the empirical and rational subject becomes a rational subject, an incarnate reasonableness. If one deliberates and chooses, one has moved to the level of the intellectual conscious, free, responsible subject that by his [or her] choices makes himself [or herself] what he [or she] is to be and his [or her] world what it is to be.[100]

Grasping the structure and operations of human consciousness, by experiencing them, provides a means of understanding our body-mind-spirit. Having experienced our body-mind-spirit, we have data about them; interpreting the data, one has an explanation of them. One has an understanding that is grounded in evidence. The evidence of our body-mind-spirit is available. As Lonergan observes:

Despite the doubts and denials of positivists and behaviorists, no one, unless some of his [or her] organs are deficient, is going to say that never in his [or her] life did he [or she] have the experience of seeing or of hearing, of touching or smelling or tasting, of imagining or perceiving, of feeling or moving; or that if he [or she] appeared to have such experience, still it was mere appearance, since all his [or her] lifelong he [or she] has gone about like a somnambulist without any awareness of his [or her] own activities.[101]

In other words, as Ogden and Richards state, to accept the material-only tenets of evidence-based research, one must be "affecting general anesthesia."[102] That is, one must be going through life with a mindless and spiritless body.

breaking through

sage body-mind-spirit

H appiness has been, and remains, a primary human aspiration. However, happiness experienced as the product of unreasonable and irresponsible choices can have catastrophic consequences and leave us in a state of alienation, misery, and despair. There is a natural path that is immune from the alienating and destructive consequences of the indiscriminate pursuit of happiness. It is a path that begins and ends at the same point. It is the path of creation, creativity, genuineness, and authenticity. It is a transcendent path that creates, conserves, and concurs with reality each and every step of the journey. It is that path from which the human mind has emerged to support the needs of every molecule, cell, tissue, and organ in our bodies, while moving us to the fullness of the unity of the universe of being. It is our sage body-mind-spirit that begins and ends with the wisdom, prudence, and good judgment built into our DNA that permeates the totality of our being.

The genuine and authentic happiness experienced as the result of reasonable and responsible actions results in an ever-deepening connectedness with others, our communities, the planet, and ourselves.

Our pursuit of Pleasure Island happiness is the primary reason our lives are difficult and full of miserable options and outcomes. We didn't get this way by delaying gratification or dedicating ourselves to healthy lifestyles, fiscal responsibility, self-sacrifice, and compromise. There is nothing new about our current unhappy situation. History is littered with lives and cultures that ended in heaps of misery and despair. The disease, while expressed by different symptoms, always has the same cause: arrogant, impulsive, self-serving actions that define what is unreasonable and irresponsible. Such is the epitaph written on every tyrant's gravestone. It is the asterisk that soils otherwise honorable and remarkable lives. It is the only enemy we have. It causes us to feel miserable. Unreasonable and irresponsible activity is the only threat we face in leading a life of genuine happiness.

We need to change course and we need to know with certainty what path will create a society and a world defined by genuine happiness. A happiness that is only realized through the creation of sustainable relationships built on reasonable and responsible activity. It is not a difficult task. It is our natural state. It is built into every molecule, cell, tissue, and organ of our bodies. It is the substance of our body-mind-spirit. It is not only in our DNA, it is our DNA. It operates in every conscious thought we have. It defines the meaning and purpose of who and what we are.

Our task is to apply our nature to each and every decision we make. Our task is to accept the momentary discomfort that comes along with reasonable and responsible living. With each and every reasonable and responsible act we perform we participate in the process of positive self-transcendence as it promotes our ever-deeper experience of the meaning and purpose of life and aligns us with the source of all that is true and good.

In living within our created nature we become deeply connected to ourselves, others, our communities, the environment and, indeed, the universe. Our journey to discover the secrets of genuine happiness ends up at its point of departure. The secret to lasting genuine happiness is found in nature. Humans are a unique expression of nature. When we act in opposition to our nature we are certain to experience the self-alienation of those actions in our body-mind-spirit. Developing patterns that conflict with our nature is certain to lead us to misery and despair.

Thus, it is not how smart we are, or the extent of our physical ability that determines our ultimate wellness and potential to experience genuine happiness. It is how we live our lives moment to moment in response to whatever we face that determines our wellness. In fact, many of the most inspirational human stories have come from individuals who have severe physical and/or mental challenges. People who become leaders who dedicate their lives and leave lasting legacies of communities striving to form a more perfect union, establish justice, ensure domestic tranquility, provide for the common defense, promote the general welfare, and secure the blessings of liberty to themselves and posterity.

To these individuals the idea of having a physical or mental challenge or making personal sacrifices for the greater good infuses them with boundless energy. Our genuine heroes have embraced the relentless impulse of our guiding nature to know the reasonable and act in accordance with its demands irrespective of personal sacrifice.

Our path to genuine happiness has been available to us from the very beginning of human existence. All we need to do is click the red ruby heels of our biological slippers together and return home to our created state. There's no big secret or magical super-human intervention needed to realize genuine happiness. The miracle is that genuine happiness is our natural state of being. Our biology is designed to receive, send, and process messages that enable us to live in harmony. Activities that support and are supported by biological and natural laws produce healthy states at any and all levels of, not only human biological structure, but the universe of biology. Activities that conflict with biological laws lead to unhealthy states.

Our mental functioning, which emerges as a biological structure from our physical biology, creates states of genuine happiness through reasonable and responsible activities. Human wellness is ultimately determined by where we find ourselves on the continuum of alienation to connectedness. Our location on the connected or alienated poles of the continuum is determined by the extent to which we act in accordance with our created nature. When we engage in activities that sustain positive connectedness, we create states of genuine happiness irrespective of the momentary discomfort our commitment to the true and good might cause.

Emergent property theory and the transcendent method offer a comprehensive and systematic understanding of the human and a comprehensive and systematic methodology for determining genuine and authentic human functioning, change, and development.

Naturopathic medicine, by embracing and working with nature is open to, and in many respects incorporates, the claims of emergent property theory and the transcendental method, both are implicit in its guiding philosophy and clinical practice.

We now have the science, methodology, and clinical options to reverse the results of our flawed, alienating, and destructive pursuit of happiness, thereby dramatically improving our health and wellness by embracing naturopathic medicine.

If we are to create lives, communities, and a planet based on the connectedness of reasonable and responsible patterns of living, we need your help. We face an incredibly difficult task. We need to overcome the fierce and brutal resistance of the powerful financial interests who profit from the EBCM system and insure that we have full access to fully accredited professionals dedicated to healthcare based on mind-body-spirit science.

We wish you and yours lives defined by genuine happiness.

medical school training

Shown below is a chart indicating the difference between conventional and naturopathic medical school training. If your conventional doctor claims to offer natural treatments ask them about their education. If they did not attend a federally and regionally accredited naturopathic medical school they are not practicing natural medicine. Nor are they practicing integrative medicine. Integrative medicine requires expertise in two distinct medical systems.

Naturopathic Medical Education Comparative Curricula

Comparing Curricula of Accredited Naturopathic Medical Schools
with Conventional Medical Schools in Hours of Training

National College of Naturopathic Medicine	Bastyr University - Naturopathic Medicine	Yale University	Johns Hopkins	Medical College of Wisconsin
Federally & Regionally Accredited Naturopathic Medical School	Federally & Regionally Accredited Naturopathic Medical School	Federally & Regionally Accredited Naturopathic Medical School	Federally & Regionally Accredited Naturopathic Medical School	Federally & Regionally Accredited Naturopathic Medical School
Basic and Clinical Sciences [1]				
1548	1639	1420	1771	1363
Clerkships and Allopathic Therapeutics [2]				
2244	1925	2891 (+thesis)	3391	2311
Naturopathic Therapeutics [3]				
588	633	0	0	0
Therapeutic Nutrition:				
144	132	0	0	0
Counseling:				
144	143	Included in psychiatry	Included in psychiatry	Included in psychiatry
Total Hours of Training:				
4668	4472	4311 (+thesis)	5162	3674

1 Anatomy, cell biology, physiology, histology, pathology, biochemistry, pharmacology, lab diagnosis,neurosciences, clinical physical diagnosis, genetics, pharmacognosy, bio-statistics, epidemiology, public health, history and philosophy, ethics, and other coursework.

2   Including lecture and clinical instruction in dermatology, family
     medicine, psychiatry, medicine, radiology, pediatrics, obstetrics,
     gynecology, neurology, surgery, ophthalmology, and clinical
     electives.

3   Including botanical medicine, homeopathy, oriental medicine,
     hydrotherapy, naturopathic manipulative therapy, ayurvedic
     medicine, naturopathic case analysis/management, naturopathic
     philosophy, advanced naturopathic therapeutics.[103]

Obviously, what jumps out is the goose egg credit-hour counts
conventional doctors receive in naturopathic therapeutics. They are
taught virtually nothing about nutrition or other critical factors that
have a pervasive impact on not only the functioning of every molecule,
cell, tissue, and organ in the body but the entirety of the human body-
mind-spirit. Nor do they receive any measurable training in counseling.
Yet primary care physicians prescribe the vast majority of psychiatric
drugs. They don't even receive training in the underlying philosophy of
their medicine. They can't because there isn't any underlying philosophy
of conventional medicine. It's an ideology. An ideology is a belief that
disregards verifiable empirical evidence and imposes its non-verifiable
claims in place of the verifiable evidence. Conventional medicine,
based on an evidence-based theory of the human, rejects the empirical
evidence that humans possess both physical and mental properties.
Rather, insisting that all science must be observable and that because
mental properties can't be observed they don't exist.

Conventional medical schools are not the gold standard in the field
of health and wellness. Conventional medicine has boxed itself into
the corner of evidence-based medicine, which is controlled by outside
financial interests focused on profits. Its "one-size-fits-all" statistics-
driven, treatment protocols have created a Whack-A-Mole approach to
wellness and a superbug future, which is bankrupting the county.

The comprehensive training received by naturopathic physicians makes a huge difference in how health and wellness is defined. The difference in training is responsible for the incredible safety record naturopathic medicine has compiled over the past 100 years in providing the most effective primary care medicine available.

appendix b

evidence-based computer
mind and spirit

EBCMs have constructed a bizarre computer model of our non-observable body-mind-spirit properties so that our body-mind-spirit properties can appear to fit the evidence-based research model.

How does EBCM turn our body-mind-spirit properties into observable material matter? Our body-mind-spirit properties are transformed into material matter by reducing them to material-only non-biological computers. Computational theory views human mind-spirit experience as material information states which exist as connected elements of material-only matter. For example, our mental experience of a dog, according to the evidence-based model is actually a grouping of connected observable material matter labeled as an "information state." A cat would be a different information

140

state constructed from a different organization of material elements. Such material information states, in computerese, are referred to as conduit metaphors or memes. Conduit metaphors or memes, as Iran-Nejad explains, function as "verbal (or symbolic) frames for holding and transporting knowledge in daily communication."[104] Thus, the images and experience created by our body-mind-spirit properties are simply the illusion of body-mind-spirit experience. According to EBCM's computation model our material mind and spirit information states can be acquired, lost, stored, retrieved, and used as needed.

In plain language this means the computer is a convenient model for defending promoting the non-biological material-only dogma of EBCM. It provides metaphors by which EBCM can suspend reality and create and defend an unbelievably profitable non-biological mono-material healthcare monopoly.

Non-biological mono-material computational models of human brain functioning generally fall into two main categories, Strong Artificial Intelligence (Strong AI) or Soft Artificial Intelligence (Soft AI). Strong AI models of human brain functioning view the brain as a form of hardware and the mind as a form of software. Consciousness is viewed as a computer-like, information-processing, material only, "head-held" device.

Strong AI models of brain functioning claim human mental operations are simply sophisticated hardware and software, which generates information-processing states. Soft artificial intelligence models have a small dose of humility. Soft AI models of brain functioning claim computational models of brain activity are limited to *simulating*, not replicating, certain computational functions of the human mind. Soft AI models concede that computer programs cannot account for subjective elements of human experience such as the mental activity of creating pre-logical insights, preferences, emotions, moral meanings, and valuations, the properties of the human mind that make humans human. The difference between strong and soft AI models of our mental and spiritual properties is that strong AI models eliminate our mental and spiritual properties while soft AI models hope our mental and spiritual properties can be eliminated with advancements in computer science at some future date.

fatal flaws in computational models: stepping in quicksand
Computational theories of our material brain structure, while offering the possibility of simulating (not replicating) an extremely limited type of mental-like activity of the human mind and spirit, face a number of challenges in developing a comprehensive and systematic explanation of human mental and spiritual functioning and the impact they have on our health, wellness, and genuine happiness. For example, computational theorists have failed to explain (a) how biology functions in the emergence of human mental and spiritual experience, (b) how semantics (meaning) can emerge from syntactically (logically) developed computer programs, and (c) how the pre-logical and multidimensional subjective experience of values and preferences can emerge from logically developed computer hardware and software. Thus, while we know computer science is a product of the human mind and the human mind only exists as a property of biology, we also know computers are not biological and, thus, computers do not have either a human mind or a human spirit.

Computational theory does not provide an explanation for the necessary role biology plays in causing the emergence of our mental and spiritual properties, experience, and activities. In fact, computational theory logically reduces mental and spiritual properties to material matter and thereby eliminates biology as a factor in human functioning. Computational theory imagines mental and spiritual functioning can be divorced from biology. Thus, as Searle argues, "one of the limitations of the computational model of the mind…is how profoundly *antibiological* it is." [105]

Second, the fact that computational systems are strictly syntactical systems (syntax is the study of the logical principles and rules for language construction) also raises the question of how the human experience of semantic meaning (semantics is the study of the meaning of language expressions), which is a core dimension of human metal activity, can emerge from the purely syntactical structure of computer systems. Computer systems, which are designed and operate within formal syntactical structural systems irrespective of their level of complexity, are insufficient to cause the emergence of semantic meaning. Searle summarizes the computational theory's semantic challenge in the following manner: Computer "Programs are entirely syntactical. Minds have semantics. Syntax is not the same as, nor is it by itself sufficient for, semantics. Therefore programs are not minds…." [106]

Thus, in the absence of explaining the semantic dimension of human mental functioning, computational theories of human mental and spiritual functioning are not simulating the structure and operations of the human mind. Computational theory is simply demonstrating the computational capabilities of syntactical systems. Moreover, while computational theories of human mental activity have demonstrated the capacity to perform computational tasks through the manipulation of syntactical symbols, such syntactical manipulations highlight, rather than resolve, the symbol-grounding problem of evidence-based, mono-material theories of human mental and spiritual functioning.

The "symbol-grounding problem" is the problem of how words, which symbolize mental activity, can be linked to their underlying and often multifaceted meaning(s). All words are symbols of the concepts and meanings assigned to objects and events created by mental activity. However, for the word to have meaning it must be connected to a mind that can grasp the mental experience symbolized by the word.

In some cases a word can mean nothing even when attached to a high-functioning mind. Examples are new words to our vocabulary or "text" symbols in our children's text messages. They simply don't compute until we uncover their meaning. The point is that words, disconnected from a mind that can assign meaning to them, are meaningless.

Attempts of EBCM to simulate human mental activity by constructing an observable-only, non-biological, material computer theory of human mental functioning, far from resolving this challenge, have only highlighted the symbol-grounding problem. To the extent computational theories imagine how mental experience can be reduced to observable-only, material bits and bytes provides a basis for explaining how mental activity might be created, stored, and retrieved in observable only mono-material software, it does not explain how stored symbols can be linked to meaning. In fact, evidence-based theorists have not come close to finding any software storage disc in the brain, let alone offering any explanation as to how software can be connected to meaning.

The problem is the following: data stored on computer software is meaningless in the absence of a human mind that can interpret the data. Moreover, when human knowledge is viewed as abstract observable-only material information bits and bytes, or static symbolic representations, stored and retrieved in the brain, the symbolic information frames are detached from the multidimensional ground data from which real human concepts and symbols arise with understanding, meaning, and purpose. For example, the concept of dog can have several meanings. In one instance a dog is a loyal pet, in another instance a dog is a threat, and in certain circumstances, a dog is a meal. Moreover, our concept of a dog is dependent on a massive amount of background information that cumulates in a dog being a dog and not a stone sculpture of a dog. The observable only, material bits and bytes are claimed to make up the "mental" representations of objects and events we encounter can only signify the end result of some unpacked internal mental process.

Therefore, Iran-Nejad argues that trying to ground material bits and bytes to their meaning amounts to "forcing one's way through a Chinese/ Chinese dictionary-go-round of constructive learning buzzwords."[107] That is to say, object-like conduit and constructive learning frames can only contain abstract meanings for those who are already familiar with the syntactical language to which they apply. Those unfamiliar with the language must pass "endlessly from one meaningless symbol or symbol-string (the definiens) to another (the definiendum), never coming to a halt on what anything meant"[108] What is needed to connect symbolism to meaning is a mind capable of grasping meaning.

The fact that syntactical systems cannot cause the emergence of semantic experience pinpoints a fundamental problem in computational-based theories of the human mind and spirit. Syntax and syntactical systems only exist as closed systems of logic (they are not non-logical or pre-logical). Such systems can only be created by a mind that possesses the capacity to grasp semantic meaning. Additionally, syntax, in and of itself, is not a property of physics, physical matter, energy, biological processes, or the processes of any natural world phenomena. Thus, syntax cannot possess the power found in real biological properties of the real biological world. Semantics, as in the human mind, cannot be caused by the operations of a syntactical structure however complex it might be. Only real biological properties of the real biological world can cause the emergence of the semantic dimension of human mental and spiritual activity. Syntactical systems only exist as abstract systems created by something like a human mind. Likewise, it is only something that possesses semantic capacity, like a human mind, that can interpret the data contained in a syntactical system. Therefore, while syntactical systems can *simulate,* not replicate a very limited number of computational operations of a human mind, they cannot explain how semantics can emerge from syntactical structures. Computational models of human mental and spiritual experience fail to explain how syntactical systems can cause the emergence of semantic meaning, how the abstract symbols can retain the meanings they represent, or how the pre-logical dimension of human mental and spiritual activity emerges and functions.

Restricted to the purely logical structure of the syntactical system within which they operate, computer systems, as indicated above, also fail to offer any explanation of the pre-logical dimension of human mental functioning. Developed within the parameters of purely logical and formal syntactical systems, computer systems cannot produce the other dimensions of human mental functioning that fall outside the scope of logic. Human knowing is not purely logical. The human mind, prior to the application of logic, configures, reconfigures or organizes and reorganizes data in order to generate knowledge, and then, and only then, applies logic to mental experience. The logic of any mental experience can only be objectified after we have conscious awareness of the mental experience. As Helminiak insists:

> *Consciousness is essentially content free, and the criteria of what is as yet unspecified cannot be logically formulated. So the functioning of consciousness cannot be logically formulated. ...consciousness does not operate by simple logical deduction. Rather, consciousness advances via leaps of creative insight, and when it does, it transforms the arena, setting up new systems in which logic then pertains.*[109]

Insights emerge from the mental activities of a mind. Once an insight emerges the mind applies logic to the insight to determine the insight's validity. Computers are incapable of generating insights. Human mental and spiritual functioning always involve dimensions of pre-logical mental experience. For example, forensic psychologists have long known the pitfalls of attempting to predict the unpredictable; human behavior. In contrast to human mental activity, the operations of computer systems are completely predictable. A fundamental difference between a human mind and a computer is that non-observable, biological minds are pre-logical and non-biological computer systems can only perform operations based on the logic of installed computer software.

Logically developed computer hardware and software cannot replicate the pre-logical dimension of a non-observable human mind. Computational theory's inability to address the pre-logical dimension of human consciousness is a major pitfall in evidence-based computer theories of the human mind and spirit.

Another insurmountable problem for EBCM computer mind and spirit theorists, tied to meaning, is the need to explain how mental understanding, mental imaging, and application of meaning to mental images can arise from the fixed logic and fixed connections of software programs. Given the fluid and contextual reality of all human experience, (we might like apple pie one moment and not like it at another time or coffee may sound great or horrible given the context of the situation), evidence-based, non-biological computer theory cannot explain how spontaneous, in-the-moment, mental and spiritual experiences can arise from fixed software made up of material-only bits and bytes incapable of generating meaning. If mental activity occurs as the result, then matching and connecting input material bits and bytes with static long-term memory software, mental functioning would be prescriptive. That is, if long-term memory comprised of connected bits and bytes exist as static bit and byte blueprints, it is difficult to explain the inconsistencies that exist between new mental experience and pre-existing bit and byte past experience held as "information states." The pre-existing bits and bytes would dictate what the new bits and bytes must be. In fact, according to Blasi, the evidence-based hypothesis that knowledge is a mono-material, observable object-like phenomenon generates "an intrinsic opposition between the structural method and its underlying philosophy [logical positivism], on one side and the reality of subjectivity and freedom, on the other" [110]

Thus, not only do computational models of human mental functioning lack a necessary biological component required for human mental experience or how semantics can emerge from syntactical systems, they are completely devoid of any explanation for what function subjectivity or conscious awareness plays in human mental experience, health, wellness, and genuine happiness.

The extent to which computational models of human mental experience have failed to account for the function that human consciousness plays in human mental functioning is apparent by the fact that computer systems do not experience anything close to human conscious experience. Blasi, for example, points out that while computer systems can simulate (not replicate) certain computational activities of the human mind, computers simulate such activities "without being aware that it is doing so, that it exists, and that it is different from non-it." [111] Therefore, as Blasi continues, "if subjectivity and consciousness exist in human beings and if the mind's structures can be divorced completely from them, then structures and structuralism [computer hardware and computer software] can provide no help in understanding subjectivity and its development." [112] This inability of computational theory to develop an adequate explanation for the subjective dimension of human mental functioning prompted Pylyshyn to suggest that:

> (I)t could turn out that consciousness is not something that can be given a computational account. Similarly certain kinds of statistical learning, aspects of ontogentic development, the effects of moods and emotions, and many other important and interesting phenomena could simply end up not being amenable to a computational account. [113]

Posner supports Pylyshyn in noting that current computational models of human mental activity are "not sufficient to explain how the brain creates and contains subjective experience."[114]

A comprehensive and systematic explanation of human mental functioning simply must include an explanation of how conscious experience informs human mental and spiritual functioning. Models of human mental and spiritual functioning that eliminate biological processes and conscious experience as necessary elements of human functioning hardly seem human at all.

Finally, even within the narrow band of human mental activity that computer systems are credited with simulating, such simulation is simulation and not replication of human mental and spiritual properties and operations. In this respect, Searle points out, "the simulation of a mental state is no more a mental state than the simulation of an explosion is itself an explosion."[115]

Programmed to pound the triangle of our body-mind-spirit into the round whole of observable, material-data-only EBCM, logical positivists continue to claim that human mental and spiritual properties can be reduced to material matter based on computational theory. However, at each stop along their journey their dependence on science fiction has intensified. Connectionism, a mono-material mental-processing theory is their point of departure—both toward a mono-material fantasy of our mental and spiritual properties and from reality.

connectionism: sinking in quicksand

According to the connectionist hypothesis, fundamental mono-material neural-processing units carry out the information processing in the brain in a similar fashion to the way computers process information.

In non-biological, mono-material connectionist theory, each non-biological, mono-material neural-processing unit receives input from other non-biological, mono-material neural-processing units, compute an output value, and subsequently send the output value to other non-biological, mono-material neuro-processing units or connected clusters of non-biological, mono-material neuro-processing units. Thus, our sensory data is reduced to neuro-processing bits then configured as "information-states."

This means that when we see a dog our non-biological, mono-material computer brain creates the dog by creating millions, if not billions, of weighted non-biological, mono-material neuro-processing units, which together produce the dog and continuously produce the dog as it goes about its dog business. Thus, if the evidence-based proponents are on to something, we know to slip our hand into a plastic bag to pick up our dog's poop to keep our neighborhood clean and neighbors happy because our computer brain is somehow activating stored dog activity programs that guide our dog activity related behavior. Amazingly, our computer brain can also activate other stored software programs that simultaneously allow us to wave to Mrs. Johnson; dodge a skateboarder; confirm that the object circling above is a hawk and not a crow; complete a verse of a limerick that had previously suffered "information state block," possibly by a computer virus; and apply pre-logical, logical, moral, emotional, and value to it all, as all of it changes moment-to-moment based largely on the semantic meaning we assign to our mental experience.

Thus, the connecting of non-biological, mono-material neurological processing-units, according to EBCM computer theory, must operate in a, as yet to be identified or located, parallel-distribution processing structure of the brain. In this computer structure multiple systems of non-biological, mono-material neurological processing-units are activated at the same time to create complex and fluid information states.

In this manner, connectionist theory argues that mental experience can be explained as the activity of non-biological, mono-material connections. However, by reducing mental states to connections of physical matter there can be no "executive or overseer" feature of our mental or spiritual, "informational state," activity. Human mental and spiritual functioning are simply computational states of connected non-biological, mono-material neurological processing-units. By making mental states purely material, not only is the overseer function of our mental and spiritual properties eliminated, the totality of our mental and spiritual properties are eliminated. Our mental and spiritual properties are unnecessary to the development of a comprehensive non-biological mono-material understanding of human health, wellness, and genuine happiness. A mono-material drug can be used to re-organize our mono-material information states or, if needed, problematic mono-material clusters can surgically removed.

Keep in mind, or as an EBCM profiteer might say, "keep in an information state," our mental and spiritual experience, such as pre-logical experiences, preferences, emotions, and valuations are not explained and have no possibility of being explained in the non-biological, mono-material computational-connectionist model.

Nonetheless, connectionist theory is the gold standard EBCM explanation of the illusion of our non-observable mental and spiritual properties and experience. That is, as connectionist theory claims, the mental messaging that differentiates the biological from the non-biological is an illusion. Thus, it is entirely possible, that given the right mono-material organization, Pinocchio, can indeed, become human and Spock can be beamed to Pleasure Island.

Connectionism provides the foundation for developing a theory of how a computer mind and spirit might function. Structural Schema Theory (SST), based on computer and connectionist theory, attempts to develop and explain how connected non-biological, mono-material bits and bytes are created, stored, retrieved and altered in our computer mind and spirit.

structural schema theory: sinking up to our neck

Structural schema theory is a natural outgrowth of computational connectionist models of mono-material brain structure and functioning. SST claims that informational states occur when an input sequence of information is matched with long-term memory traces of event-and-action information states that are somehow and somewhere stored at some yet to be identified file room in the non-biological mono-material brain. So, when you see a dog, you know it's a dog because the dog folder in your non-biological mono-material brain filing cabinet of images and concepts opens up and matches the dog you're seeing with the dog image in your file cabinet. Thus, in SST, the in-the-moment dog we see becomes an informational state through the interaction of three primary components: (a) long-term memories that are fixed non-biological mono-material connections of mental units (the prior dog); (b) external information that enters the system (the in-the-moment dog); and (c) an active, processing board (prior dog/current dog integration).

According to SST, incoming data are either assimilated into a pre-existing stored memory (prior experience of the same dog) or the pre-existing memory (prior dog) is altered to accommodate incoming data that conflicts with the existing memory (a new and different dog engage in new and different dog business). Assimilation and accommodation occur in accordance with the manner in which non-biological mono-material brain neural-processing units are connected. These weighted combinations of bits and bytes (dog types and attributes) result in behavioral dispositions or behavior (good dog-pet, bad dog, freak-out and run information state actions). Dennett summarizes the underlying structure of SST when he states, "Human consciousness is itself a huge collection of memes [dog types, etc.] (or more exactly, meme-effects in brains) that can best be understood as the operation of a *'von Neumannesque'* virtual machine *implemented* in the *parallel architecture* of a brain."[116] A von

Neumann virtual machine was an early storage retrieval computer designed by John von Neumann.

Based on the observable and quantifiable research methodology of evidence-based research, SST claims that behavior or behavioral dispositions are caused by the manner in which non-biological, mono-material neural-processing units are connected. Thus, changing the pattern of abstract neural-unit connections alters the observable behavior or behavioral dispositions of the human subject.

gaps in structural schema theory:
grasping hand above the quicksand

As indicated above, a central feature of SST is the computationally inspired connectionist notion that mental phenomenon can be reduced to some observable and measurable phenomena such as weighted connections of abstract neural-processing bits and bytes. These neural processing units are thought to be stored somewhere in the physical brain as mono-material object-like memes or conduit software strings.

The theory claims that weighted neural-processing bits and bytes exist at an intralevel (a different and distinct level of the brain) area of brain architecture. In SST the *one* in the one-to-many connections of weighted intralevel neural-processing-bits and bytes are defined as a single mental micro unit, while the *many* is defined as connected micro units that form localized macro units. Thus, in the example of a dog, a paw is a micro unit and the dog is a macro unit. In SST theory more complex connections of neural processing bits and bytes are explained by reducing them to simpler connections of neural processing bits and bytes and ultimately to a single neural processing bit—all located at the same, and as of yet, undiscovered, intralevel area of brain architecture.

Thus, SST theory suggests that both ends of mental functioning, the single neural-processing bit and the schema-producing connections of neural processing bits and bytes, are derived from undifferentiated neural processing bits and bytes located at an autonomous intralevel structure of brain architecture. In constructing human mental functioning as weighted connections of abstract neural-processing units located at some intralevel area of brain architecture, SST not only faces the same observable challenges that computational theory faces in developing a comprehensive theory of mental functioning, it magnifies those challenges.

First, if human mental experience is reducible to connections of abstract and static mental bits and bytes located at a separate information state area of the brain, it is difficult to explain how such abstract and static states could generate anything meaningful. As Bateson argues, "The explanation of mental phenomena must always reside in the ... differentiation and interaction of parts."[117] There can be no differentiation and interaction of parts in an intralevel structure composed of undifferentiated abstract neural processing bits and bytes. The emergence of preference, value, and semantics in the human mind requires in each case differentiation of substrate parts. Undifferentiated abstract neural processing bits and bytes are not capable of explaining the differentiated mental experience that defines human mental experience.

Second, like computational theory, SST's proposed intralevel explanation of mental activity also faces the difficulty of reconciling its claim of intralevel brain architecture with the biologically differentiated structure of the human brain. The SST intralevel-hypothesis of mental bit and byte storage is inconsistent with its assumption that mental activity occurs through parallel distributed processing, the claim that multi areas of the brain are simultaneously involved in creating observable mono-material "mental" images. The hypothesized parallel processing distribution is inconsistent with the notion of a psychologically autonomous intralevel area of brain structure. According to SST, the intralevel or same level network of abstract mental bits and bytes is separated from the physical properties of the brain. If mental experience results from parallel distributed processing, such distribution of brain function, as Iran Nejad and Homaifar point out, "makes more concrete sense at the physical level of the three-dimensional brain."[118]

Mental experience, following SST's intralevel hypothesis, loses its connection to the brain through the introduction of an autonomous intralevel area of brain architecture. Thus, if behavioral health grounds its understanding of human mental functioning on an autonomous intralevel structure of brain architecture, behavioral health, in effect, rejects neuroanatomy and physiology as areas of research proper to its competence.

Additionally, by constructing mental experience as static observable object-like associations of neuro-processing bits and bytes, human mental functioning, as indicated earlier, becomes prescriptive, it loses its pre-logical dimension. For example, fixed long-term memories, like data held in a computer software program, would be logically formalized connections of static neural-processing bits and bytes stored as static mental images and experience. Such logically formalized blueprints would result in prescriptive or pre-determined behavior. In such a structure we become zombies or robots, we have no creativity or spirit.

However, human functioning is anything but prescriptive. Human functioning is driven by the fluid, context-conditioned nature of in-the-moment mental functioning. Human mental functioning is largely defined by its non-prescriptive, pre-logical dimension. Thus, the pre-logical dimension of human mental functioning is incompatible with SST's notions of static memory storage.

Third, as indicated above, SST theorists have yet to identify where fixed mental bits and bytes exist in the biological brain. Long ago, Angell identified the problem of trace theory (bit and byte brain storage cabinets) in arguing that, "When we are not experiencing a sensation or an idea it is, strictly speaking, non-existent."[119]

Mental and spiritual experience is more like the atmosphere than a computer. Sunny days and rainy days appear when all the elements in the atmosphere are present to create a sunny or rainy day. No two days are identical and days are not stored in an atmospheric software program. Likewise, our mental and spiritual experience is created based on a multitude of body-mind-spirit activity which changes moment-to-moment, is not stored, and is not repeatable. In short, SST cannot explain where abstract traces of connected neural processing bits and bytes exist when they are not being experienced.

The problems confronting SST connectionism and computational theory are carried over to Evidence Validated Treatments (EVTs). In EBCM non-biological, mono-material connections are accomplished by utilizing EVTs. The EVT name has been changed to Evidence-based Treatments (EBT) because none of the treatments can be "validated" in the scientific meaning (based on fact) of validation. The change from "validation" to "based" provides lots of wiggle room. EVTs are how evidence-based dogma is employed in EBCM. Physical chemicals and other evidence-based treatments and procedures are used to change non-biological mono-material connections.

evidence validated treatments (EVTS): buried and left for dead

EVTs are developed from evidence-based research. EVTs do not and cannot address our mental or spiritual properties. In this respect, Gadamer argues, "the success of modern science [evidence-based research] rests on the fact that other possibilities for questioning are concealed by abstraction." The abstraction is the reduction of human mental and spiritual functioning to abstract material data. Richardson, et.al., echo Gadamer's concern stating that "...the kind of abstraction characteristic of the natural sciences may conceal a great deal of what is most important to us in the study of humans."[120] Thus, while evidence-based research can identify what material areas of the brain light up and what material brain chemicals are unleashed when people are shown a picture of a Twinkie or hold a pencil in their mouth, they have nothing to say about our mental-spiritual properties. Such data only shows the material products of mental-spiritual activity and thus the part is conflated with the whole producing billions of dollars.

Our body-mind-spirit determines human wellness and genuine happiness. In fact, it is precisely our mental and spiritual properties, the very human properties that EBCM eliminates, that make possible all activities undertaken in designing and conducting evidence-based research. Moreover, it is the reality of our mental and spiritual properties that, not only permeate all evidence-based double-blind studies with uncontrolled confounding variables, it is precisely our mental and spiritual properties that bias all evidence-based research before it is designed and undertaken. In this respect, as Kubacki (1984) states, "before results are interpreted, studies designed, and hypothesis formulated, researchers have committed themselves to a set of social, personal, and methodological values."[121] It is ironic then, that the very mental and spiritual properties that EBCM excludes from its research and treatments is the very human experience that accounts for any and all evidence-validated research undertaken.

The predominant value, covert and overt, of the EBCM system is profits. The EBCM system has swept our body-mind-spirit health and genuine happiness under the rug on which its safe deposit box sits. For example, Steven Brill, in his *Time* Magazine article, "Why Medical Bills are Killing Us," reported that MD Anderson Cancer Center in Houston, a nonprofit unit of the University of Texas, enjoyed an operating profit of $531 million or 26% in 2010.[122] "The president of MD Anderson, Ronald DePinho's compensation was $1,845,000 which does not include his unspecified financial ties to big pharma."[123] MD Anderson, in responding to Brill's questions about billing offered the following response, "The issues related to health care finance are complex for

patients, health care providers, payers, and government entities alike…
MD Anderson's clinical billing and collection practices are similar
to those of other major hospitals and academic medical centers."[124]
Duh. The MD Anderson response sounds a lot like Ralph Kramden's
"Homina, Homina, Homina" response when caught with his hand in
the cookie jar (Jackie Gleason, *The Honeymooners*). Managing editor of
Time magazine, Richard Stengel, commenting on Brill's article states,
"the problem with costs and profits is 'the chargemaster,' the mysterious
internal price list for products and services that every hospital in the US
keeps."[125]

The chargemaster is not the problem. The chargemaster is a
symptom of the problem. The problem, as stated above, is that EBCM is
based on the dogma of evidence-based research. Having positioned itself
as a quasi-religion, EBCM argues its evidence-based dogma can't be
questioned. Immune from questioning, the powerful EBCM profiteers,
even at non-profit institutions like MD Anderson, use their complex
statistics and complex finances to secure huge profits from consumers
and third-party payers with little concern for actual outcomes.

Computational theory, connectionism, SST, and EVTs are
underlying theories that dominate how EBCM defines and treats
the human body without consideration of the human mind-spirit.
Moreover, as a monopoly, EBCM determines what healthcare treatment
choices are available to consumers and what treatments are reimbursable
by private insurance companies and government financed programs.

EBTs provide a statistical level of certainty for the observable mono-
material data EBCM research can measure, which, in turn, provides the
bases for quantifying Whack-A-Mole treatment outcomes in bell curve
research findings. The EBCM system then moves on to the profits to
be had by treating the side effect moles that pop up each time a mole is
whacked. The process follows the consumer until the consumer declares
bankruptcy or dies.

notes

1   Kringelbach, Morten L. Web. <http://news.bbc.co.uk/2/hi/
    programmes/happiness_formula/4880272.stm>.

2   Peck, MD, M.S. *The Road Less Traveled.* New York: Simon and
    Schuster, 1978. Print.

3   19 June 2003. Web. <http://www.usgovernmentdebt.us>.

4   "Obesity Initiative." *Obesity Initiative.* Web. 22 Dec. 2014.
    <http://obesity.ovpr.uga.edu/obesity-facts/>.

5   Web. <http://blog.sparefoot.com/3230-a-brief-history-of-self-
    storage/>.

6   *Ibid.*

7   Aquinas, Thomas. *Summa Theologica.* Vol. I-II.3. Benzinger
    Brothers, 1917. Print.

8   Al-Qarni, Ayed. "Some of the Means for Achieving Happiness."
    The Religion of Islam. 23 Mar. 2009. Web. <http://www.
    islamreligion.com/articles/2407/3/23/2009>.

9   Haidt, Jonathan. *The Happiness Hypothesis: Finding Modern Truth in Ancient Wisdom*. New York: Basic, 2006. 315. Print.

10   Seligman, M. *Authentic Happiness: Using the New Positive Psychology to Realize Your Potential for Lasting Fulfillment*. New York: Free, 2002. Print.

11   Avena, N. M., P. Rada, and B. G. Hoebel. "Sugar and Fat Binging Have Notable Differences in Addictive-like Behaviors." *Journal of Nutrition* 1 Jan. 2006: 622-28. Print.

12   Lonergan, B. F. F. *Method in Theology*. New York: Herder and Herder, 1972. 20. Print.

13   Null, ND, G., M. Fieldman, MD, D. Rasio, and C. Dean, MD, ND. *Death by Medicine*. Mount Jackson: Praktikos, 2010. Print.

14   Brill, S. "Why Medical Bills Are Killing Us." *Time*. 4 Apr. 2013: 16-55. Print.

15   "Medical Waste." *Pollution Issues*. 15 Nov. 2011. Web. <http://www.pollutionissues.com/Li-Na/Medical-Waste.html>.

16   "Bryan Magee talks to A. J. Ayer about logical positivism and its legacy." *Men of Ideas*. Bryan Magee. BBC, . 1 Jan. 1978. Radio.

17   Dennett, D. *Brainstorms*. Montgomery: Bradford. 112 - 113. Print.

18   Taylor, C. *Philosophic Papers: Vol 1. Human Agency and Language*. Vol. 1. Cambridge: Cambridge UP, 1985. Print.

19   *Chicago Sun-Times*. 10 May 2013: 56. Print.

20   *Ibid*.

21   *U.S. Preventive Services Task Force*. Web. <http://www.uspreventiveservicestaskforce.org/uspstf/grades.htm>.

22   *Ibid*.

23   Carpenter, Daniel P. "The Political Economy of FDA Drug Review: Processing, Politics, And Lessons For Policy." *Health Affairs* 1 (2004): 52-63. Print.

24   *U.S. Food and Drug Administration*. Web. <http://www.fda.gov>.

25 Memorandum from Paul Leber, director, Division of
Neuropharmacological Drugs, to Robert Temple, director, Office
of New Drug Evaluation I, Subject: "NDA 20–658, Requip
[ropinerole HCl tablets]," 6–7, NDA Public File 20–658, FDA
Center for Drug Evaluation and Research.

26 McCarthy, M. (1997). *Pluralism, invariance, and conflict.*
(Bernard Lonergan on invariants of intentional subjectivity). The
Review of Metaphysics, 51(1) 3-21,p. 3

27 *Ibid.*

28 *Ibid.*

29 Messer, S.B. & Wachtel, P. L. (1997). The contemporary
psychotherapeutic landscape: Issues and prospects. In P.L.
Wachtel & S. B. Messer, (Eds.). Theories of psychotherapy:
Origins and evolution (1-27), Washington, D.C.: American
psychological Association, p.12.

30 Richardson, F. C., B. J. Fowers, and C. B. Buignon. *Re-
envisioning Psychology: Moral Dimensions of Theory and Practice.*
San Francisco: Jossey-Bass, 1999. 189. Print.

31 Pluralism, invariance, and conflict

32 Strong, MD, B. W. *Chicago Tribune.* Print.

33 Lindlahr, Henry. *Nature Cure: Philosophy and Practice Based on
Unity of Disease and Cure.* Chicago: Nature Cure, 1922. Print.

34 *Washington Association of Naturopathic Physicians.* Web. <http://
wanp.org/>.

35 *American Association of Naturopathic Physicians.* Web. <http://
www.naturopathic.org/>.

36 Mendelsohn, R. S. *How To Raise A Healthy Child... In Spite Of
Your Doctor.* New York: Ballantine, 1987. Print.

37 Searle, J. R. *The Mystery of Consciousness.* New York: NYREV,
1997. 204. Print.

38   Dunne, T. *Lonergan and Spirituality: Towards a Spiritual Integration*. Chicago: Loyola UP, 1985. 43 - 44. Print.

39   *Ibid*, p.45

40   Bateson, G. *Mind and Nature: A Necessary Unity*. New York: E.P. Dutt, 1979. 230. Print.

41   *bid*, p. 228

42   *Ibid*, p. 183

43   *Ibid*, p. 47-48

44   *Ibid*, p. 48

45   D.A. Helminiak, personal communication, August 8, 2005

46   Pert, C. D. *Molecules of Emotions*. New York: Scribner, 1999. Print.

47   *Ibid*, p. 68

48   *Ibid*, p. 185

49   *Ibid*, p. 184

50   Chopra, D. *Ageless Body, Timeless Mind*. New York: Harmony, 1993. 115. Print.

51   *Ibid*, p. 24

52   *Ibid*, p. 24

53   Searle, J. R. *The Mystery of Consciousness*. New York: NYREV, 1997. 8. Print.

54   *Ibid*, p. XIII

55   *Ibid*, p. XIV

56   Lonergan, B. F. F. *Insight: A Study of Human Understanding*. New York: Longmans, Philosophical Library, 1957. Print.

57   Bartlett, Frederic C. *Remembering; a Study in Experimental and Social Psychology,*. New York: Macmillan;, 1932. Print.

58   Helminiak, D. A. *The Human Core of Spirituality: Mind as Psyche and Spirit*. New York: State U of New York, 1996. 45 - 46. Print.

59   *Ibid*, p. 46-47

60 Lonergan, B. F. F. *Cognitional Structure. In F.E. Crowe (Ed.). Collection: Papers by Bernard Lonergan.* Montreal: Palm, 1967. 227. Print.

61 Lonergan, B. F. F. *Insight: A Study of Human Understanding.* New York: Longmans, Philosophical Library, 1957. 321. Print.

62 *Ibid*, p. 321

63 *Ibid*, p. 322

64 *Ibid*, p. 322

65 Helminiak, D. A. *The Human Core of Spirituality: Mind as Psyche and Spirit.* New York: State U of New York, 1996. 45. Print.

66 Lonergan, B. F. F. *Method in Theology.* New York: Herder and Herder, 1972. 9. Print.

67 Helminiak, D. A. *The Human Core of Spirituality: Mind as Psyche and Spirit.* Albany: New York: State U of New York, 1996. 28. Print.

68 Lonergan, B. F. F. *Insight: A Study of Human Understanding.* New York: Longmans, Philosophical Library, 1957. 322. Print.

69 *Ibid*, p. 322

70 *Ibid*, p. 323

71 Lonergan, B. F. F. *Method in Theology.* New York: Herder and Herder, 1972. 9. Print.

72 Lonergan, B. F. F. *Insight: A Study of Human Understanding.* New York: Longmans, Philosophical Library, 1957. 322. Print.

73 Helminiak, D. A., July 22, 2005, Personal Communication.

74 Lonergan, B. F. F. *Insight: A Study of Human Understanding.* New York: Longmans, Philosophical Library, 1957. 282. Print.

75 Lonergan, B. F. F. *Method in Theology.* New York: Herder and Herder, 1972. 9. Print.

76 McCarthy, M. "Pluralism, Invariance, and Conflict." *The Review of Metaphysics* 51(1).3-21 (1997): 10. Print.

77 Longmans, Philosophical Library

78 Helminiak, D. A. *The Human Core of Spirituality: Mind as Psyche and Spirit.* Albany: New York: State U of New York, 1996. 28. Print.

79 Shimoff, M. *Happy for No Reason: 7 Steps to Being Happy from the inside out.* New York: Free, 2008. Print.

80 Fukuyama, M. A. *Integrating Spirituality into Multicultural Counseling.* Thousand Oaks, 1999. Print.

81 Wolf, F. A. *The Spiritual Universe: One Physicists Vision of Spirit, Soul, Matter, and Self,.* Portsmouth: Moment Point, 1999. Print.

82 Shafranske, E. P., and R. L. Gorsuch. "Factors Associated with the Perception of Spirituality in Psychotherapy." *Journal of Transpersonal Psychology* (1984): 16, 222, 231-241. Print.

83 Elkins, D. N., L. J. Hedstrom, L. L. Hughes, J. A. Leaf, and C. Saunders. "Toward a Humanistic-phenomenological Spirituality." *Journal of Humanistic Psychology* (1988): 5-18, 28. Print.

84 Kelly, E. W. *Spirituality and Religion in Counseling and Psychotherapy: Diversity in Theory and Practice.* Alexandria: American Counseling Association, 1995. Print.

85 The Center for Human Development

86 Blasi, A. *Concept of Development in Personality Theory. In J. Loevinger, Ego Development.* San Francisco: Jossey-Bass, 1976. 29-53. Print.

87 *Ibid*, p. 43

88 McCarthy, M. "Pluralism, Invariance, and Conflict. (Bernard Lonergan on Invariants of Intentional Subjectivity)." *The Review of Metaphysics* 51(1).3-21 (1997): 5. Print.

89 Lonergan, B. F. F. *Method in Theology.* New York: Herder and Herder, 1972. Print.

90 *Ibid*, p. 23 Sillyness

91 *Ibid*, p. 4

92   *Ibid*, p. 6

93   *Ibid*, p. 6

94   *Ibid*, p. 6

95   *Ibid*, p. 6

96   *Ibid*, p. 6

97   Exner, Jr., J. E. *A Primer for Rorschach Interpretation*. Asheville: Rorschach Workshops, 2000. Print.

98   Rogers, C. R. *Actualizing Tendency in Relation to "motives" and Consciousness, In M. R. Jones (Ed.)*. Lincoln: U of Nebraska, 1963. 17. Print.

99   Helminiak, D. A. *The Human Core of Spirituality: Mind as Psyche and Spirit*. Albany: New York: State U of New York, 1996. 16. Print.

100   Lonergan, B. F. F. *Cognitional Structure. In F.E. Crowe (Ed.). Collection: Papers by Bernard Lonergan*. Montreal: Plam, 1967. 221-239. Print.

101   Lonergan, B. F. F. *Method in Theology*. New York: Herder and Herder, 1972. 16-17. Print.

102   Ogden, C. K., and I. A. Richards. *The Meaning of Meaning*. New York: Hardcourt Brace, 1923. 23. Print.

103   *Curriculum Directory of the Association of American Medical Colleges*

104   Iran-Nejad, A. "Knowledge, Self-regulation, and the Brain-mind Cycle of Reflection." *The Journal of Mind and Behavior* 21(1 & 2) (2000): 67-88. Print.

105   Searle, J. R. *The Mystery of Consciousness*. New York: NYREV,, 1997. 190. Print.

106   *Ibid*, p. 11-12

107   Harnod cited in Iran-Nejad, A. "Knowledge, Self-regulation, and the Brain-mind Cycle of Reflection." *The Journal of Mind and Behavior* 21(1&2) (2000): 67-88. Print.

108 *Ibid*, p.71
109 Helminiak, D. A. *The Human Core of Spirituality: Mind as Psyche and Spirit*. Albany: New York: State U of New York, 1996. 112-113. Print.
110 Blasi, A. *Concept of Development in Personality Theory. In J. Loevinger, Ego Development*. San Francisco: Jossey-Bass, 1976. 46. Print.
111 *Ibid*, p. 47
112 *Ibid*, p. 47
113 Pylshyn, Z. W. *Computing in Cognitive Science. In M. I. Posner (Ed.), Foundations of Cognitive Science*. Cambridge: MIT, 1993. 49-92. Print.
114 Posner, M. I. *Preface: Learning Cognitive Science. In M. I. Posner (Ed.), Foundations of Cognitive Science*. Cambridge: MIT, 1993. XIII. Print.
115 Searle, J. R. *The Mystery of Consciousness*. New York: NYREV, 1997. 18. Print.
116 Dennett, D. *Consciousness Explained*. New York: Little Brown, 1991. 210. Print.
117 Bateson, G. *Mind and Nature: A Necessary Unity*. New York: E.P. Dutt, 1979. 93. Print.
118 Iran-Nejad, A., and A. Homaifar. "The Nature of Distributed Learning and Remembering." *The Journal of Mind and Behavior* 21.1 & 2 (2000): 153-84; 169. Print.
119 Angell, J. R. *The Province of Functional Psychology*. Psychological Review, 1907. 14, 16-91. Print.
120 Gadamer, H. G., quoted in Richardson, F. C., B. J. Fowers, and C. B. Guignon. *Re-envisioning Psychology: Moral Dimensions of Theory and Practice*. San Francisco: Jossey-Bass. 222. Print.

121 Kubacki, S. R. "Applying Habermas's Theory of Communicative Action to Values in Psychotherapy." *Psychotherapy* 31.3 (1994): 463-77. Print.

122 Brill, S. "Why Medical Bills Are Killing Us." *Time* 181(8): 16-55. Print.

123 *Ibid.*

124 *Ibid.*

125 Stengel, R. "The High Cost of Care." *Time* 1 Jan. 2013: 16-85. Print.

CPSIA information can be obtained
at www.ICGtesting.com
Printed in the USA
LVOW12s1701180416

484132LV00007B/426/P